Practical Traditional
Chinese Medicine &
Pharmacology

Herbal Formulas

By
Geng Junying, Huang Wenquan,
Ren Tianchi and Ma Xiufeng

New World Press, Beijing

First Edition 1991
Third Printing 1997

ISBN 7 − 80005 − 118 − 8

Published by:
New World Press
24 Baiwanzhuang Road, Beijing, 100037, China

Distributed by:
China International Book Trading Corporation
35 Chegongzhuang Xilu, Beijing, 100044, China
P. O. Box 399, Beijing, China

Printed in the People's Republic of China

CONTENTS

i

v

Preface

This series of "Practical Traditional Chinese Medicine and Pharmacology" consists of five separate books: *Basic Theories and Principles; Acupuncture and Moxibustion; Medicinal Herbs; Herbal Formulas;* and *Clinical Experiences.* These books represent a comprehensive and systematic treatment of the theories and practices of traditional Chinese medicine and pharmacology. This series incorporates a practical approach to the study of Chinese medicine through its use of simple explanations and thorough outlines.

In the first volume, *Basic Theories and Principles,* the *Yin-Yang* and Five Elements theories are addressed as the basic philosophical elements of traditional Chinese medicine. The theories of physiology, pathology, etiology, diagnostic methodology, and syndrome differentiation in traditional Chinese medicine are explained in a discussion of the *zang-fu* organs (the internal organs) and channels-collaterals. These theories stress the importance of the appropriate holistic treatment according to an accurate diagnosis of the particular complaint. Thus the reader can learn the methods of understanding disease using the vantage point of traditional Chinese medicine and also command a knowledge of its basic theories.

The second volume, *Acupuncture and Moxibustion,* introduces techniques of acupuncture and moxibustion, commonly used acupuncture points, basic laws and methods of selecting points, and details of acupuncture treatment of the common diseases as described

1

in an appendix of typical cases. It enables the reader to learn not only acupuncture techniques for more than forty kinds of diseases and symptoms, but also methods of selecting appropriate points for different symptoms.

The third and fourth volumes, *Medicinal Herbs* and *Herbal Formulas,* provide exhaustive and practicable information on individual traditional Chinese medicinal herbs, and formulas of medicinal herbs. The former presents the theory of the Four Properties and Five Flavors of herbal drugs, the theory of ascending and descending, floating and sinking, and direction of action of medicinal herbs. Also discussed is a description of the origin, property, flavor, and classification of three hundred herbs according to their therapeutic action on diseases of specific channels, general therapeutic action, indications, dispensation of herbal prescription, and contraindications. Readers will learn in the fourth volume the original source and ingredients of one hundred fifty commonly used herbal formulas, and their therapeutic actions, indications, and contraindications. By bringing theories, methods, prescriptions, and individual herbs together, they reflect the philosophy of traditional Chinese medicine which applies treatment on the basis of syndrome differentiation. Readers will not only become acquainted with one hundred fifty commonly used herbal formulas, but also with the laws and methods of differentiating syndromes, the principles of constructing herbal prescriptions, and other aspects of traditional Chinese herbal medicine.

The fifth volume, *Clinical Experiences*, introduces therapeutic methods of treating common internal disease, gynecology, and pediatrics. It associates practical application of theories, methods, herbal formulas, and individual herbs with clinical methods. Moreover, readers can use the fifth volume to learn the basic methods of applying treatment according to syndrome differentiation using the theories of traditional Chinese medicine and pharmacology.

This series on traditional Chinese medicine has been compiled by professionals with many years of experience in teaching, scientific research, and clinical treatment. Each volume has been checked and approved by leading authorities in the field of traditional Chinese medicine and pharmacology. These books present the reader with an easy access to state of the art knowledge on Chinese traditional medicine and pharmacology. The information presented in this series is the product of years of combined research and provides a reference for beginners as well as professionals in the field of traditional medicine. At present it is rare to read English editions which completely and systematically introduce traditional Chinese medical philosophies and methodologies with such conciseness. We hope that this series is able to involve interested readers from all over the world in the development and dissemination of this ancient art for the benefit of the human race.

Professor Dong Jianhua

Director of the All-China Association of
Traditional Chinese Medicine
Advisor to the Public Health Ministry of
the People's Republic of China

Introduction

Chinese Herbal Formulas, part of the Practical Chinese Medicine and Pharmacology series, joins with two other volumes, *Medicinal Herbs* and *Clinical Experiences*, in providing practical applications of Chinese medicine. This volume combines traditional Chinese medicine theory with extensive information about the use of herbs in formula. A study of the formulas presented here will yield a better understanding of the theories and how to apply them in terms of mapping out treatment strategies and identifying herbal prescriptions for a particular disease.

Formulas are grouped by malady. Within each group, the various formulas are introduced. The following organization is adhered to throughout the book in order to facilitate reference.

1. Each formula begins with a listing of its Constituents, which includes the component herbs, their common names and Chinese *pinyin* names, as well as the quantities of each herb required.

2. Method Used section describes briefly how the formula is prepared.

3. The Functions the herbal formula performs are then listed succinctly.

4. The Indications section defines the conditions in terms of the language of traditional Chinese medicine for which the herbal formula is applicable.

5. The symptoms of the condition are listed next in the Manifestations section.

6. The Explanations section explains how the condition affects the patient's *qi*, channels and collaterals, blood, body fluids, etc.

7. The Herbs and Actions section groups the herbs according to the role they play in creating the overall effect of the formula.

8. The Applications section uses Western medical terminology to identify specific maladies against which the formula has proven effective.

9. Adjustments to the formula occasioned by special symptoms are presented in the Modifications section.

Through their mutual restraint or mutual reinforcement, herbs can fully display their actions while limiting their toxins. This has been proven by modern scientific research in China. With the aim of meeting the needs of doctors practicing tradtional Chinese medicine throughout the world, we have included in this book over one hundred representative and well-known formulas which are commonly used today. We have designed the book to be a practical, useful guide in your clinical practice. We hope it will be an effective tool in your application of traditional Chinese medicine.

I. Formulas to Release the Exterior

Formulas that promote sweating, release the exterior and encourage expulsion of rashes are called releasing exterior formulas. In this section, the formulas for treating exterior syndromes caused by exogenous pathogenic wind and cold or by exogenous pathogenic wind and heat are introduced. As for the formulas which can release the exterior syndromes resulting from invasion by exogenous pathogenic summer-heat, dryness and dampness will be introduced in an other section. Generally speaking, the formulas which can release the exterior may be divided into three categories according to their properties:

1. Releasing exterior formulas with pungent and warm properties. They dispel wind and cold and are usually used for treating exterior syndromes caused by wind and cold.

2. Releasing exterior formulas with pungent and cold properties. They dispel wind and heat and are often used for treating exterior syndromes caused by wind and heat.

3. Releasing exterior formulas with toxic properties. They strengthen the body's resistance and release the exterior and are mainly used for treating a person with a weak constitution suffering from exterior syndromes.

Cautions: A large dosage of releasing exterior formula may cause excessive sweating which is not good for the patient. At the same time, the patient treated with releasing exterior formula should avoid cold, raw, greasy, indigestible food.

MAHUANG TANG

—Decoction of Ephedra Combination

Ephedra (Mahuang)	6 g
Cinnamon twigs (Guizhi)	4 g
Apricot seed (Xingren)	9 g
Licorice (Gancao)	3 g

Method Used: The herbs are cooked by decoction.

Functions: 1. To promote sweating and release the exterior. 2. To promote the lung's function in dispersing and descending. 3. To soothe asthma.

Indications: Wind cold exterior excess syndromes due to invasion by exogenous pathogenic wind and cold.

Manifestations:	*Explanations:*
Fever	Invasion on the exterior by exogenous pathogenic wind and cold which make pores close and impair the normal function of defensive *Qi* with the result that lung *Qi* fails in its function of dispersing and descending; channels and collaterals blocked.
Chills	
No sweating	
Headache	
General pain	
Asthma	
Thin, white tongue coating	Invasion on the exterior by exogenous pathogenic wind and cold.
Pale tongue proper	
Superficial and tense pulse	

8

Herbs and Actions

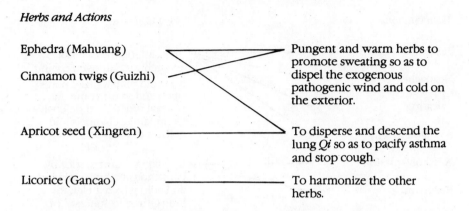

Ephedra (Mahuang)

Cinnamon twigs (Guizhi)

Pungent and warm herbs to promote sweating so as to dispel the exogenous pathogenic wind and cold on the exterior.

Apricot seed (Xingren)

To disperse and descend the lung *Qi* so as to pacify asthma and stop cough.

Licorice (Gancao)

To harmonize the other herbs.

Applications: Common cold, asthmatic bronchitis, acute rheumatic arthritis.

Modifications: 1. With asthma, cough with profuse, clear and white sputum as the main symptoms, but fever, chills, general pain and headache only mildly present. *Replace:* Cinnamon twigs (Guizhi) with Peucedanum root (Qianhu). 2. Severe arthritis. *Add:* Atractylodes rhizome (Cangzhu), Large-leaf gentiana (Qinjiao) and Honey suckle stem (Rendongteng).

GUIZHI TANG

—Decoction of Cinnamon Twigs Combination

Cinnamon twigs (Guizhi)	9 g
Licorice (Gancao)	6 g
Fresh ginger (Shengjiang)	9 g
White peony (Baishao)	9 g
Jujube (Dazao)	3 pcs

Method Used: The herbs are cooked by decoction.

Functions: 1. To promote sweating and release the exterior. 2. To harmonize the nutrient system and the defensive system.

Indications: Wind cold exterior deficiency syndromes due to weakness of the body by invasion of exogenous pathogenic wind and cold.

HERBAL FORMULAS

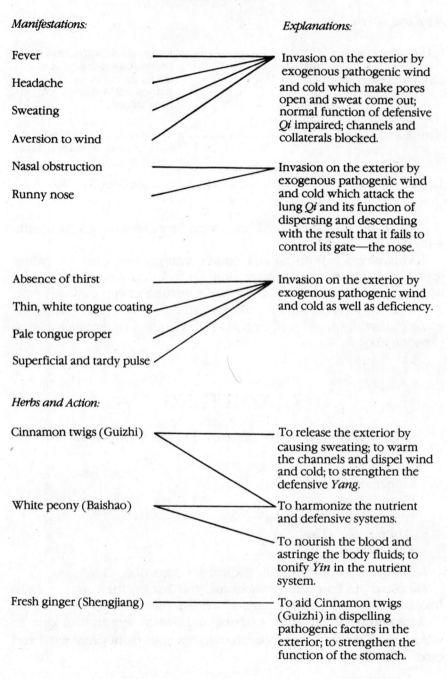

Manifestations:

Fever

Headache

Sweating

Aversion to wind

Nasal obstruction

Runny nose

Absence of thirst

Thin, white tongue coating

Pale tongue proper

Superficial and tardy pulse

Explanations:

Invasion on the exterior by exogenous pathogenic wind and cold which make pores open and sweat come out; normal function of defensive *Qi* impaired; channels and collaterals blocked.

Invasion on the exterior by exogenous pathogenic wind and cold which attack the lung *Qi* and its function of dispersing and descending with the result that it fails to control its gate—the nose.

Invasion on the exterior by exogenous pathogenic wind and cold as well as deficiency.

Herbs and Action:

Cinnamon twigs (Guizhi)

White peony (Baishao)

Fresh ginger (Shengjiang)

To release the exterior by causing sweating; to warm the channels and dispel wind and cold; to strengthen the defensive *Yang*.

To harmonize the nutrient and defensive systems.

To nourish the blood and astringe the body fluids; to tonify *Yin* in the nutrient system.

To aid Cinnamon twigs (Guizhi) in dispelling pathogenic factors in the exterior; to strengthen the function of the stomach.

10

Jujube (Dazao)	———————————	To strengthen the function of the spleen in promoting *Qi*; to aid White peony (Baishao) in nourishing the blood and *Yin*.
Licorice (Gancao)	———————————	To aid the actions of Cinnamon twigs (Guizhi) and Peony (Shaoyao); to harmonize the other herbs.

Applications: Common cold, influenza.

Modifications: Imbalance of *Yin* and *Yang*, deficiency of *Yin* and *Yang*, such as nocturnal emission, excessive dreams, cold feeling of external genitalia and deficient pulse. *Add:* Dragon's bone (Longgu) and Oyster shell (Shengmuli).

JIUWEI QIANGHUO TANG

—Decoction of Nine Ingredients with Notopterygium Root

Notopterygium root (Qianghuo)	5 g
Ligusticum (Chuanxiong)	3 g
Ledebouriella root (Fangfeng)	5 g
Angelica (Baizhi)	3 g
Atractylodes rhizome (Cangzhu)	5 g
Fresh rehmannia (Shengdihuang)	3 g
Asarum (Xixin)	1 g
Scutellaria (Huangqin)	3 g
Licorice (Gancao)	3 g

Method Used: The herbs are boiled by decoction.

Functions: 1. To promote sweating and eliminate dampness. 2. To clear interior heat.

Indications: Syndromes with interior heat and invasion by exogenous pathogenic wind, cold and dampness.

11

HERBAL FORMULAS

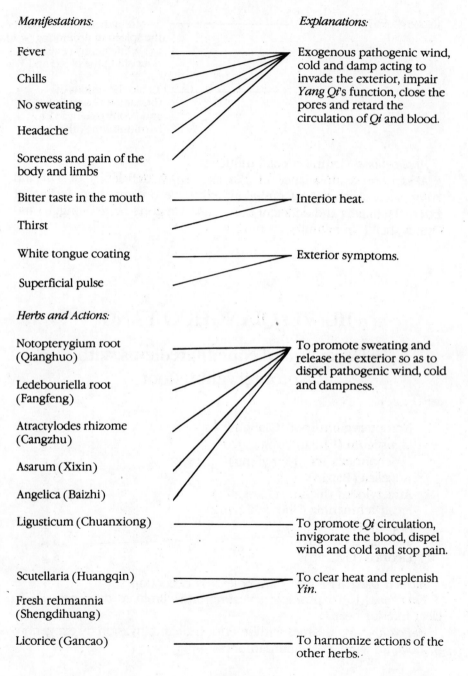

Manifestations:

Fever

Chills

No sweating

Headache

Soreness and pain of the body and limbs

Bitter taste in the mouth

Thirst

White tongue coating

Superficial pulse

Herbs and Actions:

Notopterygium root (Qianghuo)

Ledebouriella root (Fangfeng)

Atractylodes rhizome (Cangzhu)

Asarum (Xixin)

Angelica (Baizhi)

Ligusticum (Chuanxiong)

Scutellaria (Huangqin)

Fresh rehmannia (Shengdihuang)

Licorice (Gancao)

Explanations:

Exogenous pathogenic wind, cold and damp acting to invade the exterior, impair *Yang Qi*'s function, close the pores and retard the circulation of *Qi* and blood.

Interior heat.

Exterior symptoms.

To promote sweating and release the exterior so as to dispel pathogenic wind, cold and dampness.

To promote *Qi* circulation, invigorate the blood, dispel wind and cold and stop pain.

To clear heat and replenish *Yin*.

To harmonize actions of the other herbs.

12

Applications: Common cold.

Modifications: 1. Severe attack by pathogenic dampness manifested by stifling sensation in the chest. *Replace:* Fresh rehmannia (Shengdi-huang) with Bitter orange (Zhiqiao), Poria (Fuling) and Perilla leaf (Zisuye). 2. Mild soreness and pain of the body and limbs. *Delete:* Atractylodes rhizome (Cangzhu) and Asarum (Xixin). 3. No bitter taste in the mouth and thirst. *Delete:* Fresh rehmannia (Shengdihuang) and Scutellaria (Huangqin).

XIAO QINGLONG TANG

—Decoction of Minor Blue Dragon Combination

Ephedra (Mahuang)	9 g
Asarum (Xixin)	3 g
Dried ginger (Ganjiang)	3 g
Cinnamon twigs (Guizhi)	6 g
Schisandra fruit (Wuweizi)	3 g
White peony (Baishao)	9 g
Licorice (Gancao)	6 g
Pinellia tuber (Banxia)	9 g

Method Used: Ephedra (Mahuang) is first boiled and then added to the other herbs. The mixed herbs are cooked by decoction.

Functions: 1. To release the exterior and resolve phlegm fluid. 2. To stop cough and soothe asthma.

Indications: Internal retention of phlegm fluid and the exterior syndrome due to invasion by exogenous pathogenic wind and cold.

Manifestations:

Explanations:

Fever

Aversion to cold

No sweating

Invasion on the exterior by exogenous pathogenic wind and cold making pores close and depressing the *Yang Qi.*

13

Cough

Asthma

Stifling sensation in the chest

→ Lung *Qi* failing its function of dispersing and descending by retention of phlegm fluid; the exterior invaded by exogenous pathogenic wind and cold.

Dilute, white and profuse sputum

Edema on the face and limbs

→ Lung blocked by retention of phlegm fluid which is retained in the skin.

No thirst

White and watery tongue coating

→ Internal retention of phlegm fluid.

Superficial and tight pulse

→ Exterior invaded by exogenous pathogenic wind and cold.

Herbs and Actions:

Ephedra (Mahuang)

Cinnamon twigs (Guizhi)

→ To promote the lung's function in dispersing and descending so as to soothe asthma.

Asarum (Xixin)

→ To promote sweating and release the exterior.

Dried ginger (Ganjiang)

Pinellia tuber (Banxia)

→ To resolve phlegm fluid so as to stop cough and soothe asthma.

Schisandra fruit (Wuweizi)

White peony (Baishao)

→ To astringe *Yin Qi* in order to prevent the above-mentioned herbs from consuming *Qi* and *Yin*.

Licorice (Gancao)

→ To coordinate the actions of the other herbs.

Applications: Bronchitis, bronchial asthma and pulmonary emphysema.

Modifications: Heat signs of red tongue proper, irritability and rapid pulse. *Add:* Gypsum (Shigao).

JIAWEI XIANGSU SAN

—Powder of Two Effective Ingredients with Cyperus Peel and Perilla Leaf

Perilla leaf (Zisuye)	5 g
Citrus peel (Jupi)	4 g
Cyperus tuber (Xiangfu)	4 g
Baked licorice (Zhigancao)	2.5 g
Ligusticum (Chuanxiong)	1.5 g
Schizonepeta (Jingjie)	3 g
Large-leaf gentiana (Qinjiao)	3 g
Ledebouriella root (Fangfeng)	3 g
Chastetree fruit (Manjingzi)	3 g
Fresh ginger (Shengjiang)	3 slices

Method Used: The herbs are ground into powder.
Functions: To promote sweating and release the exterior.
Indications: Mild common cold due to invasion by pathogenic wind and cold.

Manifestations:

Explanations:

Fever

Chills

No sweating

Headache

Body pain

Exogenous pathogenic wind and cold acting to invade the exterior, close pores and impair the circulation of *Qi* and blood.

Nasal obstruction

Runny nose

Stifling sensation in the chest

Exogenous pathogenic wind and cold attacking the exterior and impairing the lung *Qi* in dispersing.

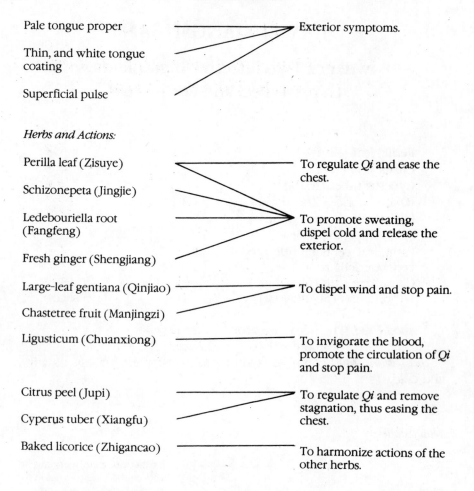

Pale tongue proper

Thin, and white tongue coating

Superficial pulse

Exterior symptoms.

Herbs and Actions:

Perilla leaf (Zisuye)

Schizonepeta (Jingjie)

Ledebouriella root (Fangfeng)

Fresh ginger (Shengjiang)

Large-leaf gentiana (Qinjiao)

Chastetree fruit (Manjingzi)

Ligusticum (Chuanxiong)

Citrus peel (Jupi)

Cyperus tuber (Xiangfu)

Baked licorice (Zhigancao)

To regulate *Qi* and ease the chest.

To promote sweating, dispel cold and release the exterior.

To dispel wind and stop pain.

To invigorate the blood, promote the circulation of *Qi* and stop pain.

To regulate *Qi* and remove stagnation, thus easing the chest.

To harmonize actions of the other herbs.

Applications: Wind-cold type of common cold in all seasons.

Modifications: 1. Cough. *Add:* Platycodon (Jiegeng), Apricot seed (Xingren) and Peucedanum root (Qianhu). 2. Sore throat. *Add:* Arctium fruit (Niubangzi) and Platycodon (Jiegeng). 3. Indigestion or epigastric fullness. *Add:* Hawthorn fruit (Shanzha), Germinated barley (Maiya) and Radish seed (Laifuzi).

XIANGRU SAN

—Decoction of Elsholtzia Combination

Elsholtzia (Xiangru)	15 g
Magnolia bark (Houpo)	12 g
Dolichos seed (Biandou)	12 g

Method Used: The herbs are ground into powder, then boiled in water with wine.

Functions: 1. To eliminate summer-heat and release the exterior. 2. To resolve dampness and harmonize the spleen and stomach.

Indications: External wind-cold syndrome, endogenous cold-damp syndrome by over-intake of cold food and drinks and prolonged exposure to cold in the summer season.

Manifestations: *Explanations:*

Fever

Chills

No sweating

Headache

Exogenous pathogenic wind and cold acting to invade the exterior, close the pores, depress the *Yang Qi* and retard the circulation of *Qi* and blood.

Stifling sensation in the chest

Vomiting

Diarrhea

Abdominal pain

Spleen and stomach injured by dampness and causing dysfunction of the organs in ascending and descending, leading to *Qi* stagnation.

Heavy sensation in the head

Lassitude and fatigue

White and sticky tongue coating

Cold and dampness in the interior.

Superficial pulse

Exterior symptoms

17

Herbs and Actions:

Elsholtzia (Xiangru)	———————— Pungent, warm and aromatic herbs to promote sweating and release the exterior so as to dispel cold, dampness and summer-heat.
Magnolia bark (Houpo)	———————— Pungent, bitter and warm herb to promote *Qi* circulation and resolve dampness.
Dolichos seed (Biandou)	———————— To strengthen the spleen and harmonize the middle *jiao* so as to remove dampness and reduce summer-heat.

Applications: Common cold, influenza and acute gastroenteritis in any season of the year.

Modifications: 1. Heat transformed from dampness accumulation manifested by thirst, irritability and yellow tongue coating. *Add:* Coptis (Huanglian). 2. Invasion of summer-heat and damp-heat in the interior manifested by fever, no sweating, slight chills, headache, stifling sensation and fullness in the chest and abdominal region, irritability, thirst, red tongue with thin and white coating and surging and big pulse. *Add:* Lonicera flower (Jinyinhua) and Forsythia (Lianqiao). This prescription is called Xinjia Xiangru Yin. 3. Severe abdominal distension and diarrhea. *Add:* Poria (Fuling), White atractylodes (Baizhu) and Plantain seed (Cheqianzi). 4. Severe chills, fever and no sweating, accompanied by nasal obstruction or runny nose. *Add:* Allium bulb (Congbai) and Prepared soybean (Dandouchi).

XINJIA XIANGRU YIN

—Decoction of Elsholtzia with Some New Herbs Added

Elsholtzia (Xiangru)	6 g
Lonicera flower (Jinyinhua)	9 g

Fresh Dolichos flower (Xian Biandouhua)	9 g
Magnolia bark (Houpo)	6 g
Forsythia (Lianqiao)	9 g

Method Used: The herbs are cooked with five cups of water resulting in two cups of liquid after decoction. Drink the hot decoction until sweat appears.

Functions: 1. To dispel summer-heat and release the exterior. 2. To clear heat and resolve dampness.

Indications: Exterior syndromes due to invasion by summer-heat, dampness and cold.

Manifestations:

Explanations:

Fever

Chills

Headache

No sweating

Exogenous pathogenic cold attacking the exterior, blocking the pores, impairing the defensive *Qi*'s function and blocking the circulation of channels and collaterals.

Thirst

Red face

Signs of excessive summer-heat.

Stifling sensation in the chest

Invasion by pathogenic dampness causing *Qi* stagnation.

White sticky tongue coating

Superficial and rapid pulse

Damp heat in the interior and the existence of the exterior symptoms.

Herbs and Actions:

Elsholtzia (Xiangru)

Pungent and warm herb to promote sweating and release the exterior.

Fresh Dolichos flower (Xian Biandouhua)

Magnolia bark (Houpo)

Fragrant herbs to resolve dampness and eliminate summer heat.

Lonicera flower (Jinyinhua) ⟶ Pungent and cool herbs to release toxins and clear heat.

Forsythia (Lianqiao)

Applications: Common cold in the summer.

Modifications: 1. Sweating and chills. *Delete:* Elsholtzia (Xiangru). 2. No stifling sensation in the chest, sticky tongue coating and symptoms due to dampness. *Delete:* Magnolia bark (Houpo). 3. Diarrhea. *Add:* White atractylodes (Baizhu), Poria (Fuling) and Plantain seed (Cheqianzi). 4. Nausea and vomiting. *Add:* Fresh ginger (Shengjiang), Bamboo shavings (Zhuru) and Pinellia tuber (Banxia). 5. Excessive heat manifested by irritability and scanty and brown urine. *Add:* Coptis (Huanglian) and Bamboo leaf (Zhuye).

SANG JU YIN

—Decoction of Mulberry Leaf and Chrysanthemum Combination

Mulberry leaf (Sangye)	7.5 g
Chrysanthemum (Juhua)	3 g
Apricot seed (Xingren)	6 g
Forsythia (Lianqiao)	5 g
Mentha (Bohe)	2.5 g
Platycodon (Jiegeng)	6 g
Licorice (Gancao)	2.5 g
Reed root (Lugen)	6 g

Method Used: The herbs are boiled with two glasses of water resulting in one glass of liquid after decoction.

Functions: 1. To dispel wind and clear heat. 2. To promote the lung's function in dispersing and descending for stopping cough.

Indications: Cough due to exogenous wind and warmth attacking the lungs.

Manifestations:

Explanations:

Cough —————————— The lung *Qi* failing its function of dispersing and descending due to the invasion of exogenous pathogenic wind and warmth.

Slight fever —————————— Slight invasion by pathogenic factors.

Slight thirst —————————— Injury of body fluids by pathogenic warmth.

Thin, white tongue coating

Superficial and rapid pulse —————————— Exterior symptoms.

Herbs and Actions:

Mulberry leaf (Sangye)

Chrysanthemum (Juhua)

Mentha (Bohe) —————————— To clear and dispel wind and heat in the upper *jiao*.

Forsythia (Lianqiao) —————————— To clear heat, release toxins and dispel wind and heat.

Platycodon (Jiegeng)

Apricot seed (Xingren) —————————— To descend the lung *Qi* so as to stop cough and resolve phlegm.

Reed root (Lugen) —————————— To clear heat and promote the production of body fluid so as to relieve thirst.

Licorice (Gancao) —————————— To harmonize actions of other herbs.

Applications: Influenza, acute bronchitis and some other upper respiratory tract infections.

Modifications: 1. Excessive heat manifested by severe cough. *Add:*

21

Anemarrhena (Zhimu) and Gypsum (Shigao). 2. Cough with yellow and thick sputum. *Add:* Trichosanthes (Gualou), Scutellaria (Huangqin) and Houttuynia (Yuxingcao). 3. Severe thirst. *Add:* Trichosanthes root (Tianhuafen). 4. Eye disorder (conjunctivitis) due to wind-heat. *Replace:* Apricot seed (Xingren) with Prunella spike (Xiakucao) and Cassia (Juemingzi). 5. Severe sore throat (acute tonsillitis). *Add:* Scrophularia (Xuanshen) and Arctium fruit (Niubangzi).

YIN QIAO SAN

—Powder of Lonicera Flower and Forsythia Combination

Forsythia (Lianqiao)	9 g
Lonicera flower (Jinyinhua)	9 g
Platycodon (Jiegeng)	6 g
Mentha (Bohe)	6 g
Prepared soybean (Dandouchi)	5 g
Bamboo leaf (Zhuye)	4 g
Licorice (Gancao)	5 g
Schizonepeta spike (Jingjiesui)	5 g
Arctium fruit (Niubangzi)	9 g
Reed root (Lugen)	9 g

Method Used: The herbs are ground into powder.

Functions: 1. To promote sweating and release the exterior. 2. To clear heat and release toxins.

Indications: Pathogenic heat in the defensive system as in the initial stage of febrile disease.

FORMULAS TO RELEASE THE EXTERIOR

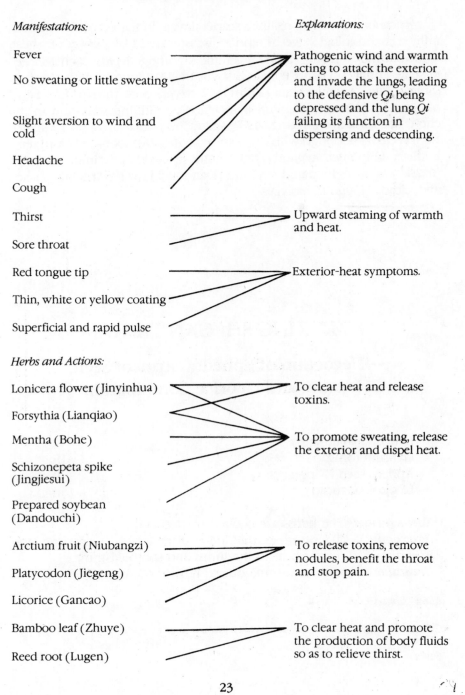

Manifestations:

Fever

No sweating or little sweating

Slight aversion to wind and cold

Headache

Cough

Thirst

Sore throat

Red tongue tip

Thin, white or yellow coating

Superficial and rapid pulse

Herbs and Actions:

Lonicera flower (Jinyinhua)

Forsythia (Lianqiao)

Mentha (Bohe)

Schizonepeta spike (Jingjiesui)

Prepared soybean (Dandouchi)

Arctium fruit (Niubangzi)

Platycodon (Jiegeng)

Licorice (Gancao)

Bamboo leaf (Zhuye)

Reed root (Lugen)

Explanations:

Pathogenic wind and warmth acting to attack the exterior and invade the lungs, leading to the defensive *Qi* being depressed and the lung *Qi* failing its function in dispersing and descending.

Upward steaming of warmth and heat.

Exterior-heat symptoms.

To clear heat and release toxins.

To promote sweating, release the exterior and dispel heat.

To release toxins, remove nodules, benefit the throat and stop pain.

To clear heat and promote the production of body fluids so as to relieve thirst.

23

Applications: Acute tonsillitis, scarlet fever, initial stage of measles, influenza and initial stage of febrile disease caused by exogenous heat.

Modifications: 1. High grade fever and sweating. *Replace:* Schizonepeta spike (Jingjiesui) and Prepared soybean (Dandouchi) with Gypsum (Shigao) and Anemarrhena (Zhimu). 2. Severe sore throat. *Add:* Scrophularia (Xuanshen) and Puff-ball (Mabo). 3. Stifling sensation in the chest, nausea and vomiting. *Add:* Agastache (Huoxiang) and Eupatorium (Peilan). 4. Cough with thick sputum. *Add:* Apricot seed (Xingren), Fritillary bulb (Beimu) and Trichosanthes (Gualou). 5. Initial stage of measles. *Replace:* Prepared soybean (Dandouchi) with Arnebia (Zicao) and Cicada slough (Chanyi).

MA XING SHI GAN TANG

—Decoction of Ephedra, Apricot Seed, Gypsum and Licorice Combination

Ephedra (Mahuang)	5 g
Gypsum (Shigao)	18 g
Apricot seed (Xingren)	9 g
Licorice (Gancao)	6 g

Method Used: The herbs are cooked by decoction.

Functions: 1. To promote the lung's function in dispersing and descending. 2. To clear heat in the lungs and soothe asthma.

Indications: Cough or asthma due to heat in the lung.

Manifestations:

Explanations:

Cough or asthma

Fever

Qi perversion caused by heat in the lungs.

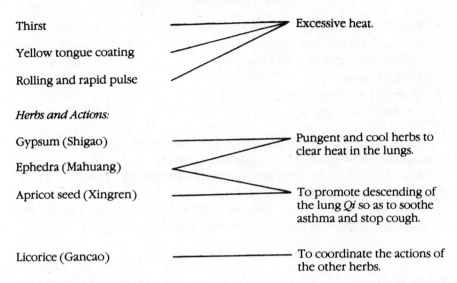

Thirst

Yellow tongue coating

Rolling and rapid pulse

Excessive heat.

Herbs and Actions:

Gypsum (Shigao)

Ephedra (Mahuang)

Pungent and cool herbs to clear heat in the lungs.

Apricot seed (Xingren)

To promote descending of the lung *Qi* so as to soothe asthma and stop cough.

Licorice (Gancao)

To coordinate the actions of the other herbs.

Applications: Lobar pneumonia, infantile pneumonia and bronchial asthma.

Modifications: 1. Sweating: The proper ratio of dosage between Ephedra (Mahuang) and Gypsum (Shigao) should be 1:5; No sweating, the ratio is 1:3. 2. Bronchial asthma. *Add:* Earthworm (Dilong). 3. Stifling sensation in the chest and cough with profuse sputum. *Add:* Lepidium seed (Tinglizi), Mulberry bark (Sangbaipi) and Trichosanthes (Gualou).

BAIDU SAN

—Powder to Release Toxins

Bupleurum (Chaihu)	30 g
Peucedanum root (Qianhu)	30 g
Ligusticum (Chuanxiong)	30 g
Bitter orange (Zhiqiao)	30 g

Ginseng (Renshen)	30 g
Notopterygium root (Qianghuo)	30 g
Pubescent angelica root (Duhuo)	30 g
Poria (Fuling)	30 g
Platycodon (Jiegeng)	30 g
Licorice (Gancao)	15 g

Method Used: The herbs are ground into powder, then boiled with Fresh ginger (Shengjiang) and Mentha (Bohe).

Functions: 1. To promote sweating and release the exterior. 2. To dispel wind and eliminate dampness.

Indications: Deficiency of anti-pathogenic factors accompanied by invasion by exogenous pathogenic wind, cold and dampness.

Manifestations:

Fever

Chills

No sweating

Stiff neck

Soreness and pain of the body and limbs

Stifling and fullness in the chest and epigastric region

Nasal obstruction

Cough with sputum

White, sticky tongue coating

Superficial, rapid pulse

Pulse being forceless even with heavy press

Explanations:

Pathogenic wind and cold acting to attack the exterior, close the pores and depress the *Yang Qi.*

Circulation of *Qi* and blood in the channels and collaterals blocked by invasion of pathogenic wind, cold and dampness.

Qi stagnation by dampness.

Exogenous pathogenic factors impairing the lung *Qi*'s function in dispersing and descending.

Excessive dampness.

Exterior symptoms.

Qi deficiency.

26

Herbs and Actions:

Notopterygium root (Qianghuo)	Pungent and warm herbs to promote sweating and dispel pathogenic wind, cold and dampness.
Pubescent angelica root (Duhuo)	
Bupleurum (Chaihu)	Pungent and cold herbs for dispersing heat.
Mentha (Bohe)	
Ligusticum (Chuanxiong)	To invigorate the blood and promote the circulation of *Qi* so as to stop pain.
Platycodon (Jiegeng)	To promote the circulation of lung *Qi* and stop cough.
Peucedanum root (Qianhu)	
Poria (Fuling)	To resolve phlegm and eliminate dampness.
Fresh ginger (Shengjiang)	
Bitter orange (Zhiqiao)	To promote *Qi* to ease the chest.
Ginseng (Renshen)	To tonify *Qi* and strengthen the body's resistance.
Licorice (Gancao)	To harmonize actions of the others herbs.

Applications: Common cold, influenza and rheumatosis.

Modifications: 1. No cough. *Replace:* Platycodon (Jiegeng), Peucedanum root (Qianhu) with Mulberry twig (Sangzhi) and Honey suckle stem (Rendongteng). 2. Initial stage of dysentery. *Replace:* Ginseng (Renshen) with Costus root (Muxiang) and Coptis (Huanglian). 3. Initial stage of boils and ulcers. *Replace:* Ginseng (Renshen) with Lonicera flower (Jinyinhua) and Forsythia (Lianqiao). 4. Severe cough. *Replace:* Notopterygium root (Qianghuo), Pubescent angelica root (Duhuo) and Ligusticum (Chuanxiong) with Pinellia (Banxia), Aster root (Ziwan) and Stemona root (Baibu).

27

JIAJIAN WEIRUI TANG

—Decoction of Polygonatum Combination

Polygonatum (Shengweirui)	9 g
Prepared soybean (Dandouchi)	9 g
Fresh allium bulb (Shengcongbai)	6 g
Platycodon (Jiegeng)	5 g
Swallowwort (Baiwei)	3 g
Mentha (Bohe)	5 g
Baked licorice (Zhigancao)	1.5 g
Jujube (Dazao)	2 pcs

Method Used: The herbs are cooked by decoction.

Functions: 1. To replenish the *Yin* and clear heat. 2. To promote sweating and release the exterior.

Indications: Yin deficiency in constitution by invasion of exogenous pathogenic wind.

Manifestations:

Fever

Slight aversion to wind and cold

Headache

No sweating or little sweating

Explanations:

Exogenous pathogenic factors acting to invade the exterior, impair the defensive *Qi*'s function and retard the circulation of *Qi* and blood.

Cough

Exogenous pathogenic factors attacking the lungs leading to the lung *Qi* failing its function of dispersing and descending.

Thirst

Dry throat

Irritability

Red tongue with scanty coating

Rapid pulse

Signs caused by *Yin* deficiency and internal heat.

28

Herbs and Actions:

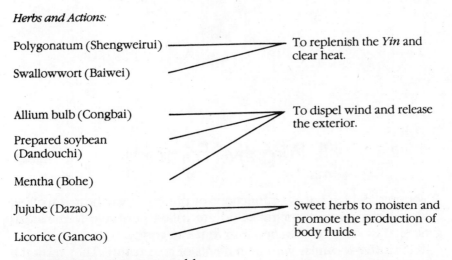

Polygonatum (Shengweirui) — To replenish the *Yin* and clear heat.

Swallowwort (Baiwei)

Allium bulb (Congbai) — To dispel wind and release the exterior.

Prepared soybean (Dandouchi)

Mentha (Bohe)

Jujube (Dazao) — Sweet herbs to moisten and promote the production of body fluids.

Licorice (Gancao)

Applications: Common cold.

Modifications: 1. Severe thirst and irritability. *Add:* Trichosanthes root (Tianhuafen) and Bamboo leaf (Zhuye). 2. Cough with thick and sticky sputum. *Add:* Trichosanthes (Gualou) and Fritillary bulb (Beimu). 3. Sore throat. *Add:* Arctium fruit (Niubangzi) and Scrophularia (Xuanshen).

II. Purgative Formulas

Formulas which have the functions of purging away heat, dispelling cold and removing water retention are called purgative formulas. In general, they may be classified into four categories:

1. Purgative formulas with ingredients of cold nature. They relax the bowels and purge away heat. They are used to treat constipation by heat accumulation.

2. Purgative formulas with ingredients of warm nature. They dispel cold and are mainly used for treating constipation by cold accumulation.

3. Purgative formulas with ingredients for moistening effects. They moisten the intestines and free bowel movements and are used to treat constipation due to dryness of the intestines.

4. Purgative formulas with ingredients for removing water retention. They remove water retention downward out of the body and are used for treating ascites and general edema.

The formulas should be used with caution in persons with weak constitutions and with pregnant women.

DA CHENGQI TANG

—Drastic Purgative Decoction

Rhubarb (Dahuang)	12 g
Magnolia bark (Houpo)	15 g
Immature bitter orange (Zhishi)	12 g
Mirabilitum (Mangxiao)	9 g

Method Used: Decoct Magnolia bark (Houpo) and Immature bitter orange (Zhishi) first, then add Rhubarb (Dahuang). When decoction is complete, add Mirabilitum (Mangxiao).

Functions: To purge the bowels and internal heat.

Indications: Excessive syndrome of the Fu organs related to Yang ming channels.

Manifestations:	*Explanations:*
Fever	Combination of heat and feces in the intestines.
Constipation	
Abdominal pain, distention and fullness	
Sensitivity to pressure on abdomen	
Dry mouth and tongue	Heat which consumes the body fluids leading to malnutrition of tendons and eyes.
Convulsion	
Blurred vision	
Yellow, thick and dry tongue coating	
Irritability	Mind disturbance by heat.
Delirium	
Cold limbs	Accumulation of heat which hinders *Yang Qi* reaching the limbs.
Deep, rolling and rapid pulse or deep, excess and forceful pulse	Signs of excess pathogenic factors in the interior.

Herbs and Actions:

Rhubarb (Dahuang)	To purge the bowels and internal heat.
Mirabilitum (Mangxiao)	

31

Magnolia bark (Houpo)

Immature bitter orange
(Zhishi)

To promote *Qi* circulation
and bowel movements and to
relieve distention and
fullness.

Applications: Appendicitis, intestinal obstruction, acute abdominal pain and high fever.

Modifications: 1. Mild damage to body fluids. *Delete:* Mirabilitum (Mangxiao). This formula is called Xiao Chengqi Tang. 2. Mild abdominal distention and fullness. *Replace:* Magnolia bark (Houpo) and Immature bitter orange (Zhishi) with Baked licorice (Zhigancao). This formula is known as Tiaowei Chengqi Tang. 3. Severe abdominal distention, fullness and pain. *Add:* Radish seed (Laifuzi), Peach seed (Taoren) and Red peony (Chishao). 4. Severe *Qi* and blood deficiency. *Add:* Ginseng (Renshen), Chinese angelica (Danggui) and Licorice (Gancao). This formula is called Huanglong Tang. 5. Severe dryness in the intestines manifested by constipation. *Replace:* Magnolia bark (Houpo) and Immature bitter orange (Zhishi) with Scrophularia (Xuanshen), Fresh rehmannia (Shengdihuang) and Ophiopogon root (Maimendong). This formula is called Zengye Chengqi Tang.

Cautions: The formula is contraindicated during pregnancy.

DAHUANG MUDANPI TANG

—Decoction of Rhubarb and Moutan Bark Combination

Rhubarb (Dahuang)	18 g
Moutan bark (Mudanpi)	9 g
Peach seed (Taoren)	12 g
Benincasa seed (Dongguazi)	30 g
Mirabilitum (Mangxiao)	9 g

Method Used: All herbs except Mirabilitum (Mangxiao) are cooked first by decoction, then the Mirabilitum (Mangxiao), decocted separately, is added to the decoction.

Functions: 1. To reduce heat and remove stagnation. 2. To disperse lumps and relieve swelling.

Indications: Initial stage of intestinal abscess.

Manifestations:

Explanations:

Right lower abdominal pain —————————— Damp-heat and stagnation of blood.

Sensitivity to pressure on the abdomen

Hard lumps

Right leg in flexed posture rather than in extended posture —————————— Extended posture of the right leg giving rise to pain.

Fever and chills —————————— Disharmony of Ying (nutrient) and Wei (defensive) systems due to accumulated heat in the blood, leading to poor circulation of *Qi* and blood.

Rolling and rapid pulse —————————— Excessive heat and dampness in the interior.

Herbs and Actions:

Rhubarb (Dahuang) —————————— To clear heat and release toxins.

To reduce heat and remove stagnation.

Mirabilitum (Mangxiao)

Moutan bark (Mudanpi) —————————— To soften hardness, disperse lumps and relieve swelling.

Peach seed (Taoren) —————————— To invigorate blood circulation, relieve swelling and stop pain.

Benincasa seed (Dongguazi) —————————— To clear heat, drain pus, eliminate dampness and relieve swelling.

33

Applications: Acute appendicitis.

Modifications: 1. Severe fever. *Add:* Lonicera flower (Jinyinhua), Dandelion (Pugongying) and Patrinia (Baijiangcao). 2. Severe pain. *Add:* Red peony (Chishao), Peach seed (Taoren) and Sichuan chinaberry (Chuanlianzi).

Cautions: The formula is contraindicated for ulcerative appendicitis and during pregnancy.

WENPI TANG

—Decoction to Warm the Spleen

Rhubarb (Dahuang)	12 g
Aconite (Fuzi)	9 g
Dried ginger (Ganjiang)	6 g
Licorice (Gancao)	3 g
Ginseng (Renshen)	9 g

Method Used: The last four ingredients are cooked with water first, then decocted Rhubarb (Dahuang) is added.

Functions: 1. To warm and tonify the spleen *Yang.* 2. To drain the cold wastes accumulation.

Indications: Constipation due to cold wastes accumulation.

Manifestations:

Constipation

Abdominal pain

Abdominal distention

Cold limbs

Chronic dysentery

Pus-like bloody stool

Explanations:

Deficiency of spleen *Yang* which leads to excessive cold and causes *Qi* stagnation.

Deficiency of spleen *Yang* which leads to excessive cold and impairs the transportation of the intestines.

White and watery tongue coating with thick coating on the root of the tongue ⟶ Signs of accumulation of cold in the interior.

Deep and tight pulse

Herbs and Actions:

Rhubarb (Dahuang) ⟶ To drain wastes accumulation.

Aconite (Fuzi) ⟶ To warm *Yang* and dispel cold.

Fresh ginger (Shengjiang) ⟶ To check the cold action of Rhubarb (Dahuang).

Ginseng (Renshen) ⟶ To tonify *Qi* in the spleen and stomach.

Licorice (Gancao)

Applications: Chronic dysentery and habitual constipation.

Modifications: 1. Severe abdominal distention and pain. *Add:* Costus root (Muxiang) and Magnolia bark (Houpo). 2. Tenesmus. *Add:* Immature bitter orange (Zhishi). 3. Severe nausea and vomiting. *Add:* Pinellia (Banxia) and Amomum (Sharen).

MAZIREN WAN

—Pills of Cannabis Seed Combination

Cannabis seed (Maziren)	500 g
White peony (Baishao)	250 g
Immature bitter orange (Zhishi)	250 g
Rhubarb (Dahuang)	500 g
Magnolia bark (Houpo)	250 g
Apricot seed (Xingren)	250 g

Method Used: The ingredients are ground into powder, then mixed with honey to make pills.

Functions: 1. To moisten the intestines and dispel heat. 2. To promote *Qi* circulation and promote bowel movements.

Indications: Constipation due to dryness and heat in the stomach and intestines.

Manifestations:	*Explanations:*
Constipation	Deficiency of body fluids due to dryness of the intestines.
Abdominal distention and fullness	*Qi* stagnation.

Herbs and Actions:

Cannabis seed (Maziren)	To nourish *Yin*, moisten dryness and promote bowel movements.
Apricot seed (Xingren)	
White peony (Baishao)	
Honey (Fengmi)	
Rhubarb (Dahuang)	To promote bowel movements and dispel heat.
Immature bitter orange (Zhishi)	To promote *Qi* circulation, relieve distention and fullness and aid bowel movements.
Magnolia bark (Houpo)	

Applications: Constipation.

Modifications: Constipation due to hemorrhoids. *Add:* Burnet root (Diyu) and Sophora flower (Huaihua).

Cautions: The formula is contraindicated during pregnancy.

SHIZAO TANG

—Decoction of Ten Jujube Combination

Genkwa (Yuanhua)	20 g
Kansui root (Gansui)	20 g

Jujube (Dazao)	10 pcs
Thistle (Daji)	20 g

Method Used: All herbs except Jujube (Dazao) are ground into powder; then 10 pieces of Jujube (Dazao) are decocted separately. The patient takes the decoction with the powder.

Functions: To drain harmful water and fluids.

Indications: Fluid retention in the hypochondrium and edema.

Manifestations:

Explanations:

1. Fluid retention in the hypochondrium:

Pain in the chest and hypochondriac region

Pain aggravated by coughing

Stifling sensation in the chest

Shortness of breath

Cannot lie flat

Fluid in the chest impairing the lung *Qi*.

Headache

Dizziness

Upward attack of harmful fluids.

Fullness and hardness in the epigastric region

Nausea

Vomiting

Upward perversion of the stomach *Qi* and fluid retention in the epigastric region.

Deep and wiry pulse

Excess pathogenic factors in the interior.

2. Edema:

General edema

Worse edema in the lower limbs

Big abdomen with distention and fullness

Abnormal defecation and urination

Retention of the harmful water which remains in the abdomen, permeates the skin, stagnates *Qi* circulation and impairs the function of the urinary bladder.

Watery tongue coating ———————— Harmful water and fluids in
the interior.

Deep, rolling and forceful
pulse

Herbs and Actions:

Thistle (Daji) ———————— To drain water and dampness
in the bowels and viscera.

Kansui root (Gansui) ———————— To drain water and dampness
in channels.

Genkwa (Yuanhua) ———————— To drain water and
dampness in the chest and
hypochondriac regions.

Jujube (Dazao) ———————— To relax the toxic actions of
the other ingredients,
promote *Qi* circulation and
protect the stomach *Qi*.

Applications: Pleurisy with effusion and edema.

Cautions: 1. The above ingredients, except Jujube (Dazao), should not be cooked, otherwise they will lose their effectiveness. 2. The formula is contraindicated during pregnancy. 3. It is also contraindicated in persons with weak constitutions.

III. Mediation Formulas

Formulas that regulate the correlations of the stomach and intestines, harmonize the spleen and liver and dispel pathogenic factors from the Shaoyang channels are called mediation formulas. In general, they can be divided into three categories:

1. Mediation Shaoyang formulas. They clear pathogenic heat and remove stagnation in the Shaoyang channels and are used for treating Shaoyang disease.

2. Formulas for regulating the function of the liver and spleen. They promote the function of the liver *Qi* in descending and dispersing and regulate the spleen *Qi*; they are also used to treat derangement of the liver and spleen.

3. Formulas for regulating the stomach and intestines. They regulate the functions of the stomach and intestines and are used to treat dysfunctions of the stomach and intestines.

XIAO CHAIHU TANG

—Decoction of Little Bupleurum Combination

Bupleurum (Chaihu)	12 g
Scutellaria (Huangqin)	9 g
Ginseng (Renshen)	6 g

Pinellia tuber (Banxia)	9 g
Licorice (Gancao)	5 g
Fresh ginger (Shengjiang)	9 g
Jujube (Dazao)	12 pcs

Method Used: The herbs are cooked twice with water by decoction.
Functions: To harmonize the Shaoyang channels.
Indications: Shaoyang syndrome.

Manifestations: *Explanations:*

Alternate chills and fever ——————— Pathogenic factor attacking Shaoyang so the struggle between the pathogenic factor and anti-pathogenic factor is carried on and gives rise to the symptom.

Stifling sensation and fullness ——————— *Qi* stagnation in the Shaoyang in the chest and channels.
hypochondriac region

Loss of appetite

Irritability ——————— Pathological change of the Shaoyang (gall bladder) affecting the stomach, leading to upward perversion of the stomach *Qi.*

Vomiting

Bitter taste in the mouth ——————— Flaring up of fire in the Shaoyang channels.

Dry throat

Dizziness

Thin, white tongue coating ——————— Pathological change of Shaoyang located between the semi-exterior and semi-interior of the body.

Wiry pulse

Herbs and Actions:

Bupleurum (Chaihu) ——————— To clear pathogenic heat and remove stagnation of *Qi* in the Shaoyang.

Scutellaria (Huangqin)

Pinellia tuber (Banxia) ——————— To conduct the perversion of *Qi* downward so as to stop vomiting.

Fresh ginger (Shengjiang)

Ginseng (Renshen)

Jujube (Dazao)

Licorice (Gancao)

To tonify *Qi* in the spleen and stomach so as to strengthen anti-pathogenic factors and dispel the pathogenic factor.

Applications: Malaria, icteric hepatitis and biliary tract inflammation.

Modifications: 1. Malaria. *Add:* Dichroa root (Changshan) and Tsaoko (Caoguo). 2. No vomiting. *Replace:* Pinellia tuber (Banxia) and Ginseng (Renshen) with Trichosanthes (Gualou). 3. Thirst. *Replace:* Pinellia tuber (Banxia) and Ginseng (Renshen) with Trichosanthes root (Tianhuafen). 4. Abdominal pain. *Replace:* Scutellaria (Huangqin) with White peony (Baishao). 5. Severe stifling sensation and fullness in the chest and epigastric region. *Add:* Cyperus tuber (Xiangfu) and Immature bitter orange (Zhishi).

DA CHAIHU TANG

—Decoction of Rhubarb and Bupleurum Combination

Bupleurum (Chaihu)	15 g
Immature bitter orange (Zhishi)	9 g
Scutellaria (Huangqin)	9 g
White peony (Baishao)	9 g
Pinellia tuber (Banxia)	9 g
Rhubarb (Dahuang)	6 g
Fresh ginger (Shengjiang)	15 g
Jujube (Dazao)	5 pcs

Method Used: The ingredients are cooked twice with water by decoction.

Functions: 1. To mediate the Shaoyang channels. 2. To reduce the accumulated heat in the interior.

Indications: Syndromes of the Shaoyang and Yangming channels.

Manifestations:

Alternate chills and fever

Fullness and stifling sensation in the chest and hypochondriac region

Nausea

Vomiting

Irritability

Fullness, hardness and pain in the epigastric region

Constipation or diarrhea

Yellow tongue coating

Wiry and forceful pulse

Herbs and Actions:

Bupleurum (Chaihu)

Scutellaria (Huangqin)

Rhubarb (Dahuang)

Immature bitter orange (Zhishi)

White peony (Baishao)

Pinellia tuber (Banxia)

Fresh ginger (Shengjiang)

Jujube (Dazao)

Explanations:

Accumulation of heat in the Shaoyang channels.

Transmission of heat from the Shaoyang to the Yangming, *Qi* stagnation and impairment of transportation in the stomach and intestines.

Excessive heat in the interior.

To clear the accumulated heat in the Shaoyang channels.

To promote bowel movements and reduce heat.

To promote *Qi* circulation, remove stagnation and relieve fullness.

To relax and stop pain.

To conduct perversion of *Qi* downward and stop vomiting.

To harmonize actions of the other herbs.

Applications: Acute cholecystitis, biliary tract stone, acute pancreatitis and intestinal obstruction.

42

Modifications: 1. Severe vomiting. *Add:* Coptis (Huanglian) and Evodia fruit (Wuzhuyu). This formula is called Zuojin Wan. 2. Jaundice. *Add:* Capillaris (Yinchenhao) and Capejasmine fruit (Zhizi). 3. Severe constipation. *Add:* Mirabilitum (Mangxiao). 4. Severe distention and fullness. *Add:* Costus root (Muxiang) and Magnolia bark (Houpo). 5. Severe pain. *Add:* Chinese angelica (Danggui) and Corydalis tuber (Yanhusuo) or Red peony (Chishao) and Peach seed (Taoren).

HAO QIN QINGDAN TANG

—Febrifugal Decoction of Sweet Wormwood and Scutellaria Combination

Sweet wormwood (Qinghao)	6 g
Bamboo shavings (Zhuru)	9 g
Pinellia tuber (Banxia)	5 g
Red poria (Chifuling)	9 g
Talc (Huashi)	9 g
Licorice (Gancao)	9 g
Scutellaria (Huangqin)	6 g
Bitter orange (Zhiqiao)	5 g
Citrus peel (Jupi)	5 g
Green Jade Powder (Biyusan)	9 g
Natural indigo (Qingdai)	9 g

Method Used: The herbs and substances are cooked with water by decoction.

Functions: 1. To clear heat and dampness in the gall bladder. 2. To harmonize the stomach and resolve phlegm.

Indications: Syndrome of excessive heat in the gall bladder channels and damp-heat in the spleen and stomach.

Manifestations:

Alternate chills and fever
(mild chills and severe fever)

Stifling sensation and fullness
in the chest and
hypochondria

Bitter taste in the mouth

Nausea

Vomiting with bitter, yellow
and sticky saliva

Red tongue with sticky
coating

Wiry, rolling and rapid pulse

Herbs and Actions:

Sweet wormwood (Qinghao)

Scutellaria (Huangqin)

Green Jade Powder
(Biyusan):
    Talc (Huashi)
    Licorice (Gancao)
    Natural indigo (Qingdai)

Red poria (Chifuling)

Bamboo shavings (Zhuru)

Pinellia tuber (Banxia)

Citrus peel (Jupi)

Bitter orange (Zhiqiao)

Explanations:

Pathogenic heat invading the
gall bladder channels and
retarding the circulation of
Qi.

Stomach affected by the
pathologic change of the gall
bladder; the spleen and
stomach obstructed by
damp-heat and the upward
perversion of the stomach *Qi*.

Excessive damp-heat in the
interior.

To clear heat and remove
stagnation in the gall bladder
channels.

To promote urination and
clear heat.

To conduct perversion of *Qi*
downward and relieve
vomiting.

To regulate *Qi* and ease the
chest.

Applications: Acute cholecystitis, acute gastritis and chronic pancreatitis.

Modifications: 1. Severe nausea and vomiting. *Add:* Coptis (Huang-lian)and Evodia fruit(Wuzhuyu).This formula is known as Zuojin Wan. 2. Jaundice. *Replace:* Citrus peel (Jupi) and Pinellia tuber (Banxia) with Oriental wormwood (Yinchen) and Capejasmine fruit (Zhizi).

JIENÜE QIBAO YIN

—Decoction of Seven Precious Ingredients to Treat Malaria

Dichroa root (Changshan)	3 g
Magnolia bark (Houpo)	1.5 g
Green tangerine peel (Qingpi)	1.5 g
Citrus peel (Jupi)	1.5 g
Baked licorice (Zhigancao)	1.5 g
Areca seed (Binglang)	1.5 g
Tsaoko seed (Caoguoren)	1.5 g

Method Used: The ingredients are cooked with water and wine by decoction and taken before a malaria attack.

Functions: 1. To dry dampness and resolve phlegm. 2. To relieve malaria.

Indications: Malaria due to phlegm heat attacking the Shaoyang channels complicated with pestilential factor.

Manifestations:	*Explanations:*
Alternate chills and fever ———————————	Pathogenic factors attacking the Shaoyang channels, and giving rise to the struggle between the anti-pathogenic factors and pathogenic factors.

White, sticky tongue coating ———————— Excessive dampness and phlegm in the interior.

Wiry and rolling pulse ———————— Qi stagnation caused by phlegm and dampness.

Herbs and Actions:

Dichroa root (Changshan) ———————— To eliminate phlegm and check the attack of malaria.

Tsaoko seed (Caoguoren) ———————— To dry dampness and eliminate phlegm.

Areca seed (Binglang)

Magnolia bark (Houpo) ———————— To promote *Qi*, remove stagnation, strengthen the spleen and resolve phlegm.

Green tangerine peel (Qingpi)

Citrus peel (Jupi)

Licorice (Gancao) ———————— To harmonize actions of the other herbs.

Applications: Malaria.

Modifications: Malaria and vomiting. *Add:* Sweet wormwood (Qinghao), Pinellia tuber (Banxia) and Fresh ginger (Shengjiang).

SINI SAN

—Four Herbs Powder to Relieve Cold Limbs

Licorice (Gancao)	6 g
Bupleurum (Chaihu)	6 g
Immature bitter orange (Zhishi)	6 g
White peony (Baishao)	9 g

Method Used: The herbs are ground into powder, or cooked by decoction.

Functions: 1. To dispel pathogenic factor and remove stagnation. 2. To regulate *Qi* in the spleen and liver.

Indications: 1. Cold limbs due to depressed liver in which the flow of *Yang Qi* is impeded. 2. Epigastric and hypochondriac pain or diarrhea from disharmony between the liver and spleen.

Manifestations:	*Explanations:*
Fever	Accumulation of heat and impairment of *Yang Qi* so that it fails to reach the hands and feet.
Cold limbs	
Epigastric and hypochondriac pain	*Qi* stagnation in the liver.
Diarrhea	Prolonged stagnation of *Qi* in the liver transforming into fire which impairs the spleen's function of transformation and transportation.
Dysentery	
Tenesmus	
Yellow tongue coating	Heat in the liver due to stagnation of *Qi* transformation.
Wiry and rapid pulse	

Herbs and Actions:

Bupleurum (Chaihu)	To clear heat and remove stagnation in the liver.
Immature bitter orange (Zhishi)	To promote *Qi* circulation and regulate the spleen and stomach.
White peony (Baishao)	To nourish blood, replenish *Yin*, pacify the liver and stop pain.
Licorice (Gancao)	To harmonize actions of the other herbs.

Applications: Liver and gall bladder disorders and stomach and intestine disorders, such as hepatitis, cholecystitis, gastritis, intercostal neuralgia, neuroses, gastric ulcer, etc.

Modifications: 1. Severe hypochondriac pain. *Add:* Curcuma root (Yujin), Cyperus tuber (Xiangfu) and Ligusticum (Chuanxiong). 2. Jaundice. *Add:* Oriental wormwood (Yinchen) and Curcuma root (Yujin).

XIAOYAO SAN

—The Ease Powder

Bupleurum (Chaihu)	30 g
Chinese angelica (Danggui)	30 g
White peony (Baishao)	30 g
White atractylodes (Baizhu)	30 g
Poria (Fuling)	30 g
Licorice (Gancao)	15 g
Mentha (Bohe)	3 g
Fresh ginger (Shengjiang)	3 g

Method Used: The herbs are ground into powder, or cooked by decoction.

Functions: 1. To promote *Qi* circulation in the liver and remove stagnation. 2. To strengthen the function of the spleen and harmonize the Ying (nutrient) system.

Indications: Disharmony between the liver and spleen, blood deficiency and stagnation of *Qi* in the liver.

Manifestations:

Costal pain

Distention in the breasts

Alternate chills and fever

Explanations:

Stagnation of *Qi* in the liver and retardation of circulation of *Qi* in the channels.

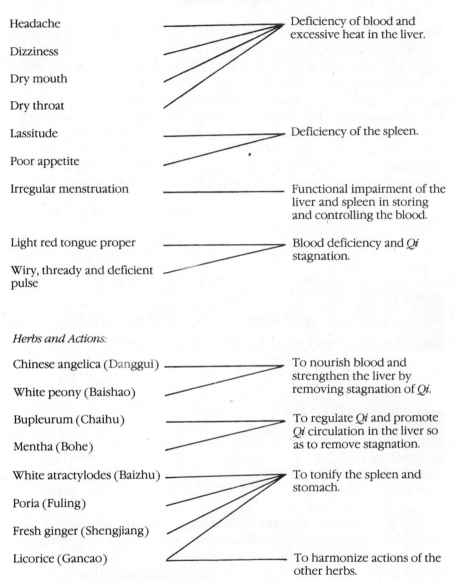

Headache

Dizziness

Dry mouth

Dry throat — Deficiency of blood and excessive heat in the liver.

Lassitude

Poor appetite — Deficiency of the spleen.

Irregular menstruation — Functional impairment of the liver and spleen in storing and controlling the blood.

Light red tongue proper

Wiry, thready and deficient pulse — Blood deficiency and *Qi* stagnation.

Herbs and Actions:

Chinese angelica (Danggui)

White peony (Baishao) — To nourish blood and strengthen the liver by removing stagnation of *Qi*.

Bupleurum (Chaihu)

Mentha (Bohe) — To regulate *Qi* and promote *Qi* circulation in the liver so as to remove stagnation.

White atractylodes (Baizhu)

Poria (Fuling)

Fresh ginger (Shengjiang) — To tonify the spleen and stomach.

Licorice (Gancao) — To harmonize actions of the other herbs.

Applications: Chronic hepatitis, neurosis, functional uterine bleeding, anemia, mastopathy and premenstrual tension.

Modifications: 1. *Qi* stagnation in the liver and blood; deficiency with heat manifested by afternoon fever, night sweating or automatic sweating; headache and red eye; palpitation, flushed malar, dry mouth; irregular menstruation and abdominal pain; bearing down sensation in the lower abdomen and difficult and painful urination. *Add:* Moutan bark (Mudanpi) and Capejasmine fruit (Zhizi). This formula is called Danzhi Xiaoyao San. 2. Severe blood deficiency. *Add:* Prepared rehmannia (Shudihuang). This formula is called Hei Xiaoyao San. 3. *Qi* deficiency. *Add:* Ginseng (Renshen) or Pilose asiabell root (Dangshen). 4. Severe costal pain. *Add:* Corydalis tuber (Yanhusuo) and Sichuan chinaberry (Chuanlianzi). 5. Red tongue and little coating. *Add:* Ligustrum fruit (Nüzhenzi), Lycium fruit (Gouqizi) and Eclipta (Hanliancao).

BANXIA XIEXIN TANG

—Decoction of Pinellia Tuber Combination to Clear Heat in the Heart

Pinellia tuber (Banxia)	9 g
Scutellaria (Huangqin)	6 g
Dried ginger (Ganjiang)	6 g
Ginseng (Renshen)	6 g
Licorice (Gancao)	6 g
Coptis (Huanglian)	3 g
Jujube (Dazao)	4 pcs

Method Used: The herbs are cooked with water by decoction.

Functions: 1. To harmonize the stomach and conduct the perversion of *Qi* downward. 2. To relieve nodules, fullness and distention.

Indications: Disharmony of the stomach *Qi* caused by damp-heat in the interior manifested in epigastric fullness and distention.

Manifestations:	*Explanations:*
Epigastric fullness and distention	*Qi* stagnation in the middle *jiao.*

Nausea

Vomiting

Borborygmus

Diarrhea

⟶ Ascending and descending functions of the spleen and stomach impaired, resulting in turbid dampness due to *Qi* stagnation in the spleen and stomach.

Thin, yellow and sticky coating ⟶ Damp-heat in the interior.

Wiry and rapid pulse ⟶ Prolonged accumulation of heat.

Herbs and Actions:

Pinellia tuber (Banxia)

Dried ginger (Ganjiang)

⟶ Pungent and hot herbs to remove nodules and stagnation.

Coptis (Huanglian)

Scutellaria (Huangqin)

⟶ Bitter and cold herbs to clear heat, dry dampness and conduct fire downward.

Ginseng (Renshen)

Jujube (Dazao)

Licorice (Gancao)

⟶ To tonify *Qi* in the spleen and stomach so as to strengthen the anti-pathogenic factors.

Applications: Acute and chronic gastritis, enteritis and indigestion.

Modifications: 1. Severe fullness and distention in the epigastric region. *Replace:* Ginseng (Renshen) with Immature bitter orange (Zhishi). 2. No weak constitution. *Replace:* Ginseng (Renshen) and Jujube (Dazao) with Citron (Xiangyuan), Finger citron (Foshou) and Magnolia flower (Xinyihua).

IV. Formulas for Clearing Heat

Formulas composed of cool and cold herbs that act to clear heat, release toxins, cool blood and treat interior heat syndromes are called clearing heat formulas. They can be classified into six categories:

1. Formulas for clearing heat in the *Qi* system. They clear heat and conduct fire downward and are used to treat heat in the *Qi* system.

2. Formulas for clearing heat and cooling blood in the Ying (nutrient) and Xue (blood) systems. They clear heat, cool blood and release toxins and are used to treat heat in the Ying (nutrient) and Xue (blood) systems.

3. Heat-clearing and detoxifying formulas. They clear heat, reduce fire and release toxins, and are used to treat syndromes caused by excessive fire and toxic heat.

4. Formulas for clearing heat in the bowels and viscera. They clear heat and release toxins and are used to treat syndromes caused by heat in the bowels and viscera.

5. Formulas for clearing heat and eliminating summer-heat. They clear heat and eliminate summer-heat and are used to treat syndromes caused by invasion of pathogenic summer-heat.

6. Formulas for clearing heat due to *Yin* deficiency. They replenish *Yin* and clear heat and are used to treat *Yin* deficiency with internal heat syndromes.

BAIHU TANG

—Decoction of White Tiger Gypsum Combination

Gypsum (Shigao)	30 g
Licorice (Gancao)	3 g
Anemarrhena (Zhimu)	9 g
Oryza (Jingmi)	9 g

Method Used: The herbs and substances are cooked with water by decoction.

Functions: To clear heat and promote the production of body fluids.

Indications: Excessive heat in the Yangming channels or excessive heat in the *Qi* systems.

Manifestations:

High fever

Irritability

Thirst

Flushed face

Profuse sweating

Dry mouth and tongue

Surging, big and forceful pulse

Explanations:

Body fluids consumed because of excessive heat in the *Qi* system.

Herbs and Actions:

Gypsum (Shigao)

Anemarrhena (Zhimu)

Oryza (Jingmi)

Licorice (Gancao)

To clear heat, replenish *Yin* and relieve thirst and irritability.

To tonify *Qi*, and prevent bitterness and cold of the first two herbs from injuring the stomach.

53

Applications: High fever in febrile diseases and diabetes.

Modifications: 1. Big and forceless pulse. *Add:* Ginseng (Renshen). 2. Swelling and pain of joints. *Add:* Cinnamon twigs (Guizhi) or Atracty-lodes rhizome (Gangzhu). 3. Compulsion. *Add:* Uncaria stem (Gouteng), Earthworm (Dilong) and Antelope's horn (Lingyangjiao).

ZHUYE SHIGAO TANG

—Decoction of Bamboo Leaf and Gypsum Combination

Bamboo leaf (Zhuye)	15 g
Gypsum (Shigao)	30 g
Ginseng (Renshen)	15 g
Ophiopogon root (Maimendong)	9 g
Licorice (Gancao)	5 g
Oryza (Jingmi)	15 g
Pinellia tuber (Banxia)	9 g

Method Used: The oryza should be cooked in the decoction made from the other herbs and substances. Then the cooked oryza should be removed from the decoction.

Functions: 1. To clear heat and promote the production of body fluids. 2. To tonify *Qi* and harmonize the stomach.

Indications: Deficiency of *Qi* and body fluids due to febrile diseases in which the remaining heat is not eliminated.

Manifestations:

Low grade fever

Profuse sweating

Irritability

Explanations:

Caused by the remaining heat.

54

Dry mouth

Thirst

Shortness of breath

Lassitude ———————————— Deficiency of *Qi* and body fluids.

Nausea

Vomiting ———————————— Upward perversion of the stomach *Qi*.

Restlessness

Insomnia ———————————— Mind disturbed by the attack of heat.

Red tongue with little coating

Deficient and rapid pulse ———————————— Deficiency of *Qi* and body fluids as well as existence of the remaining heat.

Herbs and Actions:

Bamboo leaf (Zhuye)

Gypsum (Shigao) ———————————— To clear heat and relieve irritability.

Ginseng (Renshen)

Ophiopogon root (Maimendong)

Oryza (Jingmi) ———————————— To tonify *Qi* and promote the production of body fluids.

Licorice (Gancao)

Pinellia tuber (Banxia) ———————————— To conduct *Qi* downward so as to relieve vomiting.

Applications: Children's fever in summer and late stage of febrile diseases in which *Qi* and body fluids are not restored.

Modifications: 1. Severe hot sensations of the body. *Add:* Lonicera flower (Jinyinhua) and Forsythia (Lianqiao). 2. Febrile disease in the late stage of warmth with *Yin* deficiency and internal heat remaining. *Replace:* Pinellia tuber (Banxia) with Sweet wormwood (Qinghao), Moutan bark (Mudanpi), Fresh rehmannia (Shengdihuang) and Tortoise shell (Biejia).

QINGYING TANG

—Decoction to Dispel Pathogenic Heat from *Yin* System

Rhinoceros horn (Xijiao)	2 g
Fresh rehmannia (Shengdihuang)	15 g
Red sage root (Danshen)	6 g
Coptis (Huanglian)	5 g
Lonicera flower (Jinyinhua)	9 g
Ophiopogon root (Maimendong)	9 g
Scrophularia (Xuanshen)	9 g
Bamboo leaf (Zhuye)	3 g
Forsythia (Lianqiao)	6 g

Method Used: The herbs and substances are boiled with eight glasses of water resulting in three glasses of decoction.

Functions: 1. To dispel pathogenic heat from Ying (nutrient) system. 2. To nourish *Yin* and invigorate blood.

Indications: Syndrome of pathogenic heat entering the Ying (nutrient) system.

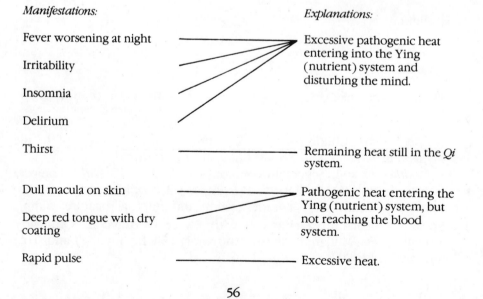

Manifestations:

Fever worsening at night

Irritability

Insomnia

Delirium

Thirst

Dull macula on skin

Deep red tongue with dry coating

Rapid pulse

Explanations:

Excessive pathogenic heat entering into the Ying (nutrient) system and disturbing the mind.

Remaining heat still in the *Qi* system.

Pathogenic heat entering the Ying (nutrient) system, but not reaching the blood system.

Excessive heat.

Herbs and Actions:

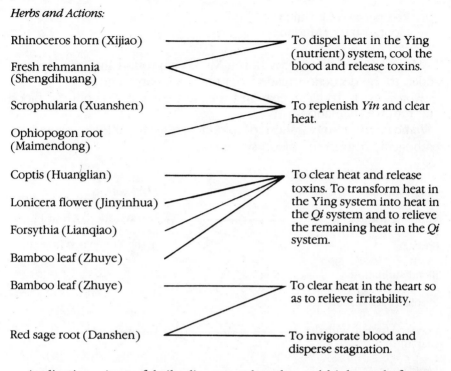

Rhinoceros horn (Xijiao)

Fresh rehmannia (Shengdihuang)

To dispel heat in the Ying (nutrient) system, cool the blood and release toxins.

Scrophularia (Xuanshen)

Ophiopogon root (Maimendong)

To replenish *Yin* and clear heat.

Coptis (Huanglian)

Lonicera flower (Jinyinhua)

Forsythia (Lianqiao)

Bamboo leaf (Zhuye)

To clear heat and release toxins. To transform heat in the Ying system into heat in the *Qi* system and to relieve the remaining heat in the *Qi* system.

Bamboo leaf (Zhuye)

To clear heat in the heart so as to relieve irritability.

Red sage root (Danshen)

To invigorate blood and disperse stagnation.

Applications: Acute febrile disease and prolonged high grade fever.

Modifications: 1. Phlegm. *Add:* Bamboo juice (Zhuli). 2. Coma. *Add:* Antelope's horn (Lingyangjiao) and Earthworm (Dilong), or use Zixue Dan or Angong Niuhuang Wan or Zibao Dan.

Cautions: The formula is contraindicated in a person with white and watery tongue coating.

XIJIAO DIHUANG TANG

—Decoction of Rhinoceros Horn and Rehmannia Combination

Rhinoceros horn (Xijiao)	1.5-3 g
Fresh rehmannia (Shengdihuang)	30 g

Red peony (Chishao)   12 g
Moutan bark (Mudanpi)   9 g

Method Used: Rhinoceros horn (Xijiao) is ground into powder and added to the decoction made from the other three herbs.

Functions: 1. To clear heat and release toxins. 2. To cool the blood and remove stagnation.

Indications: Extravasation of blood syndrome due to exogenous pathogenic heat in the blood system.

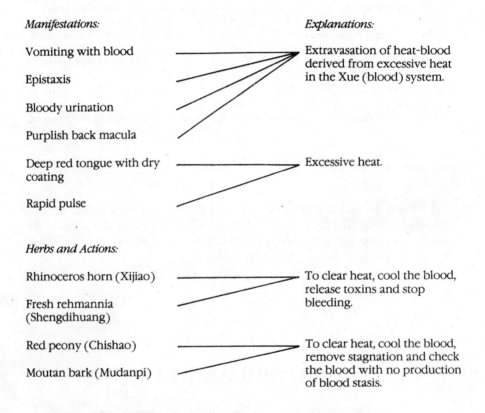

Manifestations:

Vomiting with blood

Epistaxis

Bloody urination

Purplish back macula

Deep red tongue with dry coating

Rapid pulse

Explanations:

Extravasation of heat-blood derived from excessive heat in the Xue (blood) system.

Excessive heat.

Herbs and Actions:

Rhinoceros horn (Xijiao)

Fresh rehmannia (Shengdihuang)

Red peony (Chishao)

Moutan bark (Mudanpi)

To clear heat, cool the blood, release toxins and stop bleeding.

To clear heat, cool the blood, remove stagnation and check the blood with no production of blood stasis.

Applications: Epidemic hemorrhagic fever, typhus fever, acute icteric hepatopathy, septicemia, thrombocytopenic purpura and some other hemorrhagic diseases caused by heat in the blood.

Modifications: 1. Severe vomiting with blood and epistaxis. *Add:*

Imperata rhizome (Baimaogen), Biota tops (Cebaiye) and Eclipta (Han-liancao). 2. Severe blood stool. *Add:* Burnet root (Diyu) and Sophora flower (Huaihua). 3. Severe uremia. *Add:* Small thistle (Xiaoji) and Imperata rhizome (Baimaogen). 4. Coma and convulsion. *Add:* The patent medicines, Angong Niuhuang Wan or Zixue Dan or Zibao Dan.

HUANGLIAN JIEDU TANG

—Decoction of Coptis Combination to Release Toxins

Coptis (Huanglian)	3-9 g
Scutellaria (Huangqin)	6 g
Phellodendron (Huangbai)	6 g
Capejasmine fruit (Zhizi)	9 g

Method Used: The herbs are cooked by decoction.
Functions: To reduce fire and release toxins.
Indications: Excessive toxic heat syndromes.

Manifestations: *Explanations:*

Fever —————————————— Excessive heat.

Irritability

Insomnia   Mind disturbed by excessive heat.

Cloudy mind

Epistaxis

Vomiting with blood   Extravasation of the blood caused by fire or heat.

Macula

Jaundice —————————————— Accumulation of damp-heat.

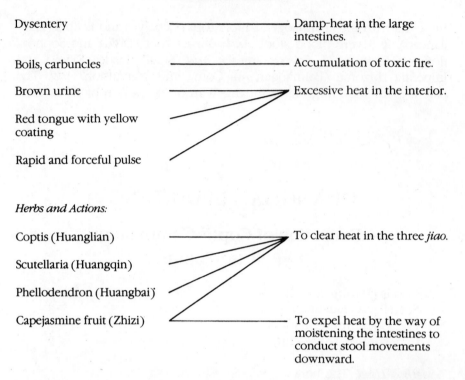

Dysentery ———————— Damp-heat in the large intestines.

Boils, carbuncles ———————— Accumulation of toxic fire.

Brown urine

Red tongue with yellow coating

Rapid and forceful pulse

Excessive heat in the interior.

Herbs and Actions:

Coptis (Huanglian)

Scutellaria (Huangqin)

Phellodendron (Huangbai)

Capejasmine fruit (Zhizi)

To clear heat in the three *jiao*.

To expel heat by the way of moistening the intestines to conduct stool movements downward.

Applications: Acute enteritis, acute dysentery, acute icteric hepatitis, septicemia, acute cholecystitis, acute pelvic inflammation, erysipelas, boils and carbuncles.

Modifications: 1. Jaundice. *Add:* Oriental wormwood (Yinchen) and Rhubarb (Dahuang). 2. Vomiting blood, epistaxis. *Add:* Imperata rhizome (Baimaogen) and Biota tops (Cebaiye). 3. Severe macula. *Add:* Moutan bark (Mudanpi) and Fresh rehmannia (Shengdihuang). 4. Red tongue and no coating. *Add:* Scrophularia (Xuanshen), Fresh rehmannia (Shengdihuang) and Ophiopogon root (Maimendong). 5. Constipation. *Add:* Rhubarb (Dahuang).

PUJI XIAODU YIN

—Universal Anti-Toxin Decoction

Scutellaria (Huangqin)	15 g
Coptis (Huanglian)	15 g
Citrus Peel (Jupi)	6 g
Licorice (Gancao)	6 g
Scrophularia (Xuanshen)	6 g
Bupleurum (Chaihu)	6 g
Isatis root (Banlangen)	3 g
Platycodon (Jiegeng)	6 g
Forsythia (Lianqiao)	3 g
Puff-ball (Mabo)	3 g
Arctium fruit (Niubangzi)	3 g
Mentha (Bohe)	3 g
White stiff silkworm (Jiangcan)	2 g
Cimicifuga (Shengma)	2 g

Method Used: The herbs are cooked by decoction.
Functions: 1. To dispel wind. 2. To clear heat and release toxins.
Indications: Epidemic febrile disease with flushed swollen face and head due to invasion by exogenous pathogenic heat and toxic factors.

Manifestations:	*Explanations:*
Fever	Dysfunction of defensive *Qi* and depression of *Yang Qi* derived from exogenous pathogenic wind heat and toxic factors invading the exterior.
Chills	
Flushed swollen face and head	Epidemic wind and heat accumulating in the upper *jiao*, and then attacking the face and head.
Sore throat	
Thirst and dry throat	Injury of body fluids by heat.

Red tongue with white or yellow coating ———————— Excessive heat.

Superficial, rapid and forceful pulse ———————— The exterior attacked by exogenous pathogenic wind and heat.

Herbs and Actions:

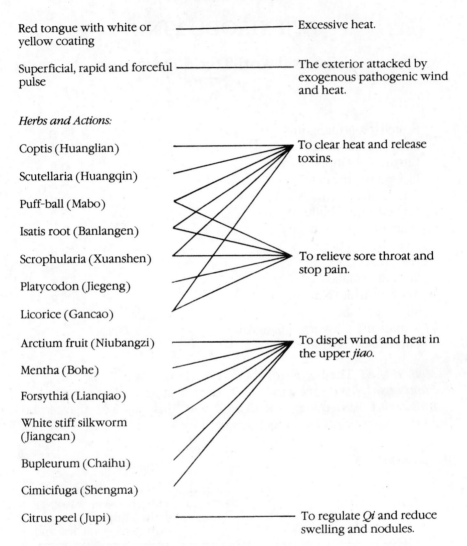

Coptis (Huanglian)

Scutellaria (Huangqin)

Puff-ball (Mabo)

Isatis root (Banlangen)

Scrophularia (Xuanshen)

Platycodon (Jiegeng)

Licorice (Gancao)

Arctium fruit (Niubangzi)

Mentha (Bohe)

Forsythia (Lianqiao)

White stiff silkworm (Jiangcan)

Bupleurum (Chaihu)

Cimicifuga (Shengma)

Citrus peel (Jupi)

To clear heat and release toxins.

To relieve sore throat and stop pain.

To dispel wind and heat in the upper *jiao*.

To regulate *Qi* and reduce swelling and nodules.

Applications: Carbuncles, furuncles, boils and swelling on face and head, epidemic parotitis, acute tonsillitis and acute submaxillary lymphadenitis

Modifications: 1. No chill. *Delete:* Mentha (Bohe) and Bupleurum (Chaihu). 2. Severe chills. *Add:* Schizonepeta (Jingjie) and Ledebouriella root (Fangfeng). 3. Constipation. *Add:* Rhubarb (Dahuang). 4. Parotitis and testitis. *Add:* Sichuan chinaberry (Chuanlianzi) and Chinese gentiana (Longdancao).

XIANFANG HUOMING YIN

—Decoction of Fairy Formula for Life

Angelica (Baizhi)	3 g
Fritillary bulb (Beimu)	3 g
Ledebouriella root (Fangfeng)	3 g
Red peony (Chishao)	3 g
Trichosanthes root (Tianhuafen)	3 g
Fresh Chinese angelica root (Shengdangguiwei)	3 g
Mastic (Ruxiang)	3 g
Lonicera flower (Jinyinhua)	9 g
Licorice (Gancao)	3 g
Gleditsia spine (Zaojiaoci)	3 g
Anteater scales (Chuanshanjia)	3 g
Citrus peel (Jupi)	9 g
Myrrh (Moyao)	3 g

Method Used: The herbs are cooked with water and wine by decoction.

Functions: 1. To clear heat and release toxins. 2. To reduce swelling and nodules. 3. To invigorate the blood and stop pain.

Indications: Initial stage of boils, carbuncles and swelling due to excess of toxic heat and stagnation of *Qi* and blood.

Manifestations:	*Explanations:*
Red swelling, hot sensation and pain in the affected area	Accumulation of toxic heat and stagnation of *Qi* and blood.

Fever, chills ———————————— Accumulation of toxic heat causing disharmony between nutrient and defensive systems.

Thin, white tongue coating or ——————— Symptoms of the initial stage slightly yellow coating of boils and carbuncles.

Rapid and forceful pulse ——————— Excess of toxic heat and vigorous anti-pathogenic factors.

Herbs and Actions:

Lonicera flower (Jinyinhua) ———————— To clear heat and release toxins.

Licorice (Gancao)

Fresh Chinese angelica root ———————— To invigorate the circulation (Shengdangguiwei) of blood and resolve stagnation for reducing Red peony (Chishao) swelling and stopping pain.

Mastic (Ruxiang)

Myrrh (Moyao)

Anteater scales ————————— To promote festering to drain (Chuanshanjia) pus.

Gleditsia spine (Zaojiaoci)

Ledebouriella root ————————— Pungent herbs to remove (Fangfeng) stagnation and harmonize the nutrient and defensive Angelica (Baizhi) systems.

Fritillary bulb (Beimu) ————————— To clear heat and release toxins and nodules.

Trichosanthes root (Tianhuafen)

Citrus peel (Jupi) ————————— To promote the circulation of *Qi* and release nodules.

Applications: Carbuncles, furuncles, boils and mastitis.
Modifications: 1. Mild pain. *Delete:* Mastic (Ruxiang) and Myrrh (Mo-

yao). 2. Severe swelling and pain. *Replace:* Ledebouriella root (Fangfeng) and Citrus peel (Jupi) with Dandelion (Pugongying) and Forsythia (Lianqiao). 3. Constipation. *Add:* Rhubarb (Dahuang).

Cautions: This formula is contraindicated in *Yin* type of boils or ulcers.

WUWEI XIAODU YIN

—The Releasing Toxins Decoction of Five Ingredients

Lonicera flower (Jinyinhua)	20 g
Wild chrysanthemum (Yejuhua)	15 g
Semiaquillegia seed (Zibei Tiankui)	15 g
Dandelion (Pugongying)	15 g
Viola (Zihuadiding)	15 g

Method Used: The herbs are cooked by decoction. Then add one or two spoonfuls of wine for boils and carbuncles.

Functions: To clear heat and release toxins.

Indications: Various swelling, boils, carbuncles and furuncles due to accumulation of toxic heat.

Manifestations: *Explanations:*

Hot sensation, swelling and pain in the affected area ——————— Accumulation of toxic heat making *Qi* and blood stagnate.

A shape like a grain of millet with a hard base, or hard as a nail is formed.

Fever

Red tongue with yellow coating ——————— Excessive toxic heat.

Rapid pulse

Herbs and Actions:

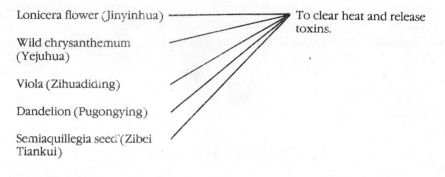

Lonicera flower (Jinyinhua)

Wild chrysanthemum (Yejuhua)

Viola (Zihuadiding)

Dandelion (Pugongying)

Semiaquillegia seed (Zibei Tiankui)

To clear heat and release toxins.

Applications: Furuncles, carbuncles, boils, erysipelas, cellulitis acute mastitis, pyogenic cholangitis, septicemia and hard inflammation.

SIMIAO YONGAN TANG

—Decoction with Four Excellent Ingredients for Carbuncle

Lonicera flower (Jinyinhua)	90 g
Scrophularia (Xuanshen)	90 g
Chinese angelica (Danggui)	30 g
Licorice (Gancao)	15 g

Method Used: The herbs are cooked by decoction.

Functions: 1. To clear heat and release toxins. 2. To invigorate the circulation of blood and stop pain.

Indications: Gangrene of the extremities (thromboangiitis) due to retardation of circulation of blood in the channels by excessive toxic fire in the interior.

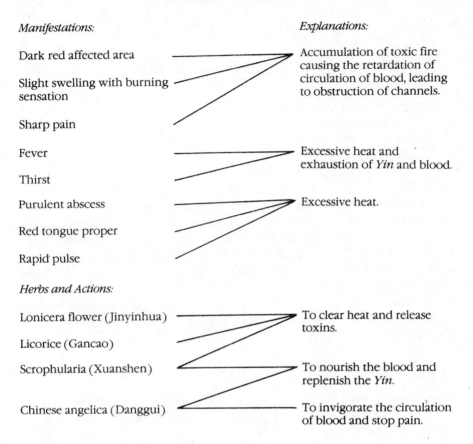

Manifestations:

Dark red affected area

Slight swelling with burning sensation

Sharp pain

Explanations:

Accumulation of toxic fire causing the retardation of circulation of blood, leading to obstruction of channels.

Fever

Thirst

Excessive heat and exhaustion of *Yin* and blood.

Purulent abscess

Red tongue proper

Rapid pulse

Excessive heat.

Herbs and Actions:

Lonicera flower (Jinyinhua)

Licorice (Gancao)

To clear heat and release toxins.

Scrophularia (Xuanshen)

To nourish the blood and replenish the *Yin.*

Chinese angelica (Danggui)

To invigorate the circulation of blood and stop pain.

Applications: Thromboangiitis.

Modifications: 1. Excessive heat. *Add:* Forsythia (Lianqiao) and Moutan bark (Mudanpi). 2. Severe pain. *Add:* Red sage root (Danshen), Mastic (Ruxiang) and Myrrh (Moyao). 3. Severe thirst. *Add:* Anemarrhena (Zhimu) and Fresh rehmannia (Shengdihuang). 4. Purplish skin on the affected area. *Add:* Peach seed (Taoren) and Carthamus (Honghua). 5. Severe distention and swelling of the affected area. *Add:* Phellodendron (Huangbai), Atractylodes rhizome (Cangzhu) and Achyranthes (Niuxi). 6. Severe purulent infection and deficiency of *Qi* and blood. *Add:* Astragalus (Huangqi), Pilose asiabell root (Dangshen) and Prepared rehmannia (Shudihuang).

Cautions: The formula is contraindicated in cold type of gangrene manifested by cold feeling with no swelling on the affected area.

XIHUANG WAN

—Pills of Bos Calculus

Bos calculus (Niuhuang)	15 g
Musk (Shexiang)	75 g
Mastic (Ruxiang)	500 g
Myrrh (Moyao)	500 g
Yellow rice (Huangmifan)	350 g

Method Used: The steamed and baked yellow rice is made into powder, then mixed with the powder made of the other ingredients and water to make pills which are then dried in a shady place.

Functions: 1. To release toxins and relieve carbuncles. 2. To resolve phlegm and remove nodules. 3. To invigorate the circulation of blood and eliminate stagnation.

Indications: Breast carcinoma, bubo, scrofula, subcutaneous nodules and multiple abscesses by stagnation of phlegm-fire or toxic heat accumulation.

Manifestations: *Explanations:*

Red tongue   Signs of stagnation of
                                     phlegm-fire
Rapid, rolling pulse

Herbs and Actions:

Bos calculus (Niuhuang) ——————— To clear heat and release
                                     toxins; to resolve phlegm and
                                     remove nodules.

Musk (Shexiang) ——————— To invigorate the blood and
                                     remove nodules, and to
                                     strengthen the action of Bos
                                     calculus (Niuhuang) in
                                     resolving phlegm.

Mastic (Ruxiang)   To invigorate blood, reduce
                                     swelling and stop pain.
Myrrh (Moyao)

Yellow rice (Huangmifan) ———————————— To prevent the other herbs
from injuring the stomach.

Applications: Lymphadenitis, multiple abscesses, mastitis and adeno-
carcinoma of the breast.
Cautions: It is contraindicated in the presence of ulceration.

DAOCHI SAN

—Powder of Fresh Rehmannia and Clematis Stem to Conduct the Fire Downward

Fresh rehmannia (Shengdihuang)	10 g
Clematis stem (Mutong)	10 g
Licorice (Gancao)	10 g
Bamboo leaf (Zhuye)	10 g

Method Used: The herbs are ground into powder.
Functions: 1. To clear heat in the heart and replenish *Yin.* 2. To
promote urination.
Indications: Painful urination or ulceration of the oral cavity due to
excessive heat in the heart channels.

Manifestations:

Explanations:

Ulceration of the oral cavity ——————————— Flaring up of fire in the heart.
and tongue

Thirst

Red face

Irritability

Fever

Frequent urination — Fire in the heart shifting into the small intestines.

Painful urination

Urgent urination

Lower abdominal distension

Red tongue proper — Signs of excessive heat.

Rapid pulse

Herbs and Actions:

Fresh rehmannia (Shengdihuang) — To clear heat, cool blood and replenish *Yin*.

Bamboo leaf (Zhuye) — To promote urination and conduct heat downward.

Clematis stem (Mutong)

Licorice (Gancao) — To reduce fire and stop pain.

Applications: Acute urinary tract infection and ulceration of the oral cavity.

Modifications: 1. Severe ulceration of the mouth and tongue. *Add:* Coptis (Huanglian). 2. Severe urinary tract infection. *Add:* Small thistle (Xiaoji), Capejasmine fruit (Zhizi) and Plantain seed (Cheqianzi).

LONGDAN XIEGAN TANG

—Decoction of Chinese Gentiana Combination to Purge Liver Fire

Chinese gentiana (Longdancao)	6 g
Scutellaria (Huangqin)	9 g

Capejasmine fruit (Zhizi)	9 g
Alisma (Zexie)	12 g
Clematis stem (Mutong)	9 g
Plantain seed (Cheqianzi)	9 g
Chinese angelica (Danggui)	3 g
Fresh rehmannia (Shengdihuang)	9 g
Bupleurum (Chaihu)	6 g
Licorice (Gancao)	6 g

Method Used: The herbs are cooked by decoction.

Functions: 1. To clear excessive fire in the liver and gall bladder. 2. To clear damp-heat in the lower *jiao*.

Indications: Flaring up of fire in the liver and gall bladder, or damp-heat in the lower *jiao*.

Manifestations: *Explanations:*

Bitter taste in the mouth   Excessive fire in the liver and
                                                      gall bladder attacking the
Red, swelling pain in the eye   head, eyes and ears along the
                                                      corresponding meridians, or
Swollen ear   stagnation of *Qi* in the liver
                                                      and gall bladder impairing
Tinnitus   the meridians.

Deafness

Headache

Hypochondriac pain

Swelling or itching in the   Damp-heat in the liver and
genital organs   gall bladder flowing along
                                                     their meridians down to the
Yellow leukorrhea   genital organs.

Turbid urine

Painful urination

Red tongue proper   Signs of excessive damp-heat.

Yellow and sticky coating

Wiry, rolling and rapid pulse

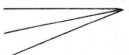

Herbs and Actions:

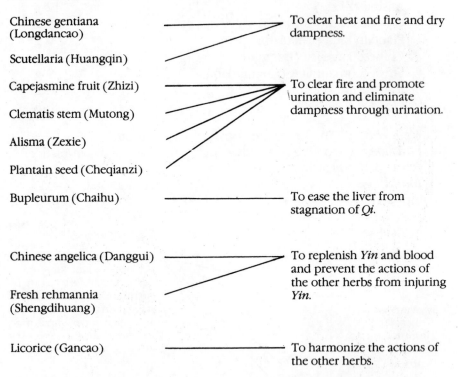

Chinese gentiana (Longdancao)

Scutellaria (Huangqin)

To clear heat and fire and dry dampness.

Capejasmine fruit (Zhizi)

Clematis stem (Mutong)

Alisma (Zexie)

Plantain seed (Cheqianzi)

To clear fire and promote urination and eliminate dampness through urination.

Bupleurum (Chaihu)

To ease the liver from stagnation of *Qi.*

Chinese angelica (Danggui)

Fresh rehmannia (Shengdihuang)

To replenish *Yin* and blood and prevent the actions of the other herbs from injuring *Yin.*

Licorice (Gancao)

To harmonize the actions of the other herbs.

Applications: Acute conjunctivitis, acute media otitis, acute icteric hepatitis, acute cholecystitis, hypertension, acute urethritis, acute prostatitis, orchitis, acute pelvic inflammation and swollen genital organs.

Modifications: Icteric hepatitis. *Replace:* Plantain seed (Cheqianzi) and Alisma (Zexie) with Oriental wormwood (Yinchen).

Cautions: It is contraindicated in a patient with red tongue with scanty coating.

ZUOJIN WAN

—Pills of Coptis and Evodia Fruit

Coptis (Huanglian)	180 g
Evodia fruit (Wuzhuyu)	15-30 g

Method Used: The powder of the herbs is made into pills.
Functions: 1. To clear fire in the liver. 2. To descend the perversion of *Qi* and stop vomiting.
Indications: Stomach attacked by liver fire.

Manifestations:

Explanations:

Hypochondriac distention and pain ———————— Stagnation of *Qi* in the liver impairing the circulation of the meridians of the liver.

Nausea, vomiting and acid regurgitation

Belching

Stagnation of *Qi* of the liver turning into fire which attacks the stomach and makes stomach *Qi* go upward.

Dry mouth ———————— Body fluids consumed by heat.

Red tongue with yellow coating

Wiry and rapid pulse

Signs of fire transformed from stagnation of *Qi* in the liver.

Herbs and Actions:

Coptis (Huanglian) ———————— Bitter and cold herb to clear heat and fire.

Evodia fruit (Wuzhuyu) ———————— Pungent and hot herb to ease the liver, descend the perversion of *Qi* and stop vomiting.

Applications: Acute and chronic gastritis.

Modifications: 1. Disharmony between the liver and stomach manifested by stomach ache, vomiting, acid regurgitation, abdominal pain, diarrhea or dysentery. *Add:* White peony (Baishao). 2. Damp-heat dysentery manifested by abdominal pain, bloody stool and tenesmus. *Add:* Costus root (Muxiang).

XIEQING WAN

—Balls to Purge the Green (Liver)

Chinese angelica (Danggui)	30 g
Chinese gentiana (Longdancao)	30 g
Ligusticum (Chuanxiong)	30 g
Capejasmine fruit (Zhizi)	30 g
Rhubarb (Dahuang)	30 g
Notopterygium root (Qianghuo)	30 g
Ledebouriella root (Fangfeng)	30 g

Method Used: The herbs are processed into balls.

Functions: 1. To clear excessive heat in the liver. 2. To conduct dampness and heat downward.

Indications: Congestion, swelling and pain of the eye caused by liver fire.

Manifestations: *Explanations:*

Congestion, swelling and   ——————————   Eye attacked by liver fire.
pain of the eye

Irritability

Hot temper   Soul disturbed by liver fire
                                             which is depressed in the
                                             interior.
Insomnia

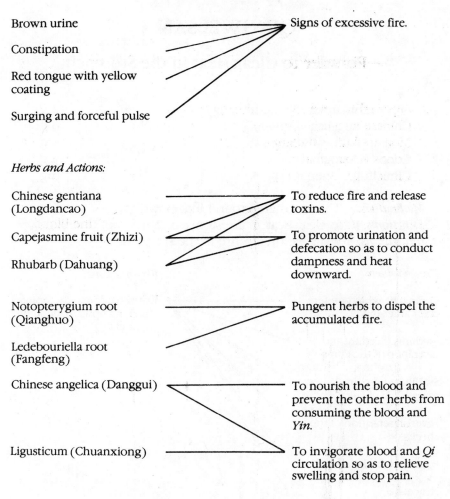

Brown urine

Constipation

Red tongue with yellow coating

Surging and forceful pulse

Signs of excessive fire.

Herbs and Actions:

Chinese gentiana (Longdancao)

Capejasmine fruit (Zhizi)

Rhubarb (Dahuang)

To reduce fire and release toxins.

To promote urination and defecation so as to conduct dampness and heat downward.

Notopterygium root (Qianghuo)

Ledebouriella root (Fangfeng)

Pungent herbs to dispel the accumulated fire.

Chinese angelica (Danggui)

To nourish the blood and prevent the other herbs from consuming the blood and *Yin.*

Ligusticum (Chuanxiong)

To invigorate blood and *Qi* circulation so as to relieve swelling and stop pain.

Applications: Eye disorders.

Modifications: In certain cases of eye disorders. *Replace:* Notopterygium root (Qianghuo), Ledebouriella root (Fangfeng) and Chinese angelica (Danggui) with Chrysanthemum (Juhua), Forsythia (Lianqiao), Fresh rehmannia (Shengdihuang) and Red peony (Chishao).

QINGWEI SAN

——Powder to Clear Heat in the Stomach

Fresh rehmannia (Shengdihuang)	12 g
Chinese angelica (Danggui)	6 g
Moutan bark (Mudanpi)	9 g
Coptis (Huanglian)	3-5 g
Cimicifuga (Shengma)	6 g

Method Used: The herbs are ground into powder.
Functions: 1. To clear heat in the stomach. 2. To cool the blood.
Indications: Toothache due to fire in the stomach.

Manifestations:

Toothache which prefers
cold rather than heat

Swelling, bleeding and
ulceration of the gums

Swelling and pain on lips,
tongue and cheeks

Feverish sensation of the
checks

Foul smell in the mouth

Headache

Red tongue with yellow
coating

Rolling and rapid pulse

Explanations:

Excessive fire in the stomach
attacking upward along the
channels.

Signs of excessive heat.

Herbs and Actions:

Coptis (Huanglian)

Cimicifuga (Shengma)

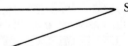

To clear heat, release toxins
and remove nodules.

Fresh rehmannia
(Shengdihuang) ——————————→ To clear heat and cool the
blood.

Moutan bark (Mudanpi)

Chinese angelica (Danggui) ————————— To nourish the blood,
invigorate blood circulation
and relieve swelling.

Applications: Stomatitis, periodontitis and trigeminal neuralgia.

Modifications: 1. Gum bleeding. *Add:* Achyranthes (Niuxi). 2. Severe swollen gum. *Add:* Lonicera flower (Jinyinhua).

YUNÜ JIAN

—The Fair Maiden Decoction of Rehmannia and Gypsum Combination

Gypsum (Shigao)	15-30 g
Prepared rehmannia (Shudihuang)	9-30 g
Ophiopogon root (Maimendong)	6 g
Anemarrhena (Zhimu)	4.5 g
Achyranthes (Niuxi)	4.5 g

Method Used: The herbs are cooked by decoction.

Functions: To clear heat in the stomach and replenish *Yin.*

Indications: Toothache caused by excessive fire in the stomach and *Yin* deficiency in the kidneys.

Manifestations: *Explanations:*

Gingival swelling, pain and ——————————→ Excessive stomach fire
bleeding   traveling along the channels
                                                                     to the upper part of the body.

Headache

Hot feeling due to irritability

Thirst

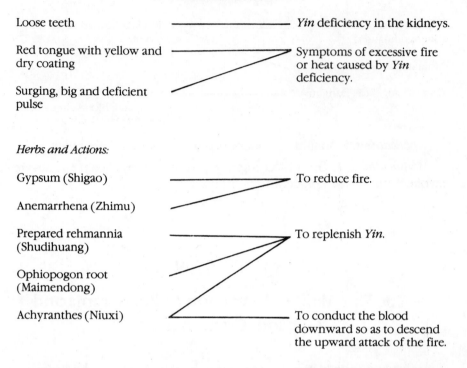

Loose teeth ———————————— *Yin* deficiency in the kidneys.

Red tongue with yellow and dry coating

Surging, big and deficient pulse

Symptoms of excessive fire or heat caused by *Yin* deficiency.

Herbs and Actions:

Gypsum (Shigao)

Anemarrhena (Zhimu)

To reduce fire.

Prepared rehmannia (Shudihuang)

Ophiopogon root (Maimendong)

Achyranthes (Niuxi)

To replenish *Yin*.

To conduct the blood downward so as to descend the upward attack of the fire.

Applications: Periodontitis and acute stomatitis.

Modifications: Severe gingival swelling, bleeding and ulceration. *Replace:* Prepared rehmannia (Shudihuang) with Fresh Rehmannia **(Shengdihuang), Moutan bark (Mudanpi), Imperata rhizome (Bai-maogen) and Eclipta (Hanliancao).**

WEIJING TANG

—Decoction of Phragmites Stem Combination

Phragmites stem (Weijing)	30 g
Coix seed (Yiyiren)	30 g
Benicasa seed (Dongguazi)	24 g
Peach seed (Taoren)	9 g

Method Used: The herbs are cooked by decoction.

Functions: 1. To clear heat in the lungs and resolve phlegm. 2. To dispel pus.

Indications: Lung abscess due to accumulation of stagnation of blood and heat-phlegm in the lungs.

Manifestations:	*Explanations:*
Cough with yellow, bloody and odorous sputum	Lungs failing their function in dispersing and descending due to excessive heat associated with phlegm, pus and stagnation of blood.
Dull pain in the chest, especially while coughing	Retardation of circulation of *Qi* and blood by stagnated phlegm and blood.
Red tongue proper with yellow coating	Signs of excessive heat and phlegm.
Rolling and rapid pulse	

Herbs and Actions:

Phragmites stem (Weijing)	To clear heat in the lungs for the treatment of lung abscess.
Benincasa seed (Dongguazi)	To dispel phlegm and pus.
Coix seed (Yiyiren)	To drain dampness and clear heat.
Peach seed (Taoren)	To invigorate blood circulation and remove stagnation.

Applications: Lung abscess, lobar pneumonia, bronchitis and bronchiectasis.

Modifications: 1. Severe heat. *Add:* Scutellaria (Huangqin), Capejasmine fruit (Zhizi), Houttuynia (Yuxingcao), Lonicera flower (Jinyinhua) and Licorice (Gancao). 2. Cough with profuse sputum. *Add:* Platycodon (Jiegeng), Apricot seed (Xingren), Tendrilled fritillary bulb (Chuanbeimu), Plantain seed (Cheqianzi) and Talc (Huashi). 3. Severe cough with bloody sputum. *Add:* Imperata rhizome (Baimaogen), Lotus node (Oujie) and Ophicalcite (Huaruishi). 4. Constipation. *Add:* Rhubarb (Dahuang).

XIEBAI SAN

—Powder to Purge the White (Lungs)

Wolfberry bark (Digupi)	30 g
Mulberry bark (Sangbaipi)	30 g
Licorice (Gancao)	30 g

Method Used: A handful of Oryza (Jingmi) is mixed with the powder of the herbs and cooked by decoction.

Functions: 1. To clear heat in the lungs. 2. To stop cough and soothe asthma.

Indications: Cough due to consuming of *Yin* by heat in the lungs.

Manifestations:	Explanations:
Cough Asthma	Upper perversion of lung *Qi* due to dysfunction of the lungs in descending.
Hot sensation of the skin No sweating	Heat in the lungs, as the lungs dominate skin and hair.
Afternoon fever	Active lung in the afternoon producing strong heat which consumes *Yin* in the lungs.
Red tongue with yellow coating	Excessive heat.
Thready and rapid pulse	Deficiency of *Yin* and body fluids.

Herbs and Actions:

Mulberry bark (Sangbaipi) ————————— To reduce heat in the lungs to stop cough and asthma.

Wolfberry bark (Digupi) ————————— To clear heat caused by *Yin* deficiency.

Oryza (Jingmi) ————————— To promote *Qi* to strengthen the stomach.

Licorice (Gancao)

Applications: Bronchitis, whooping cough, infantile pneumonia and pulmonary tuberculosis.

Modifications: 1. Severe heat manifestations. *Add:* Scutellaria (Huangqin), Anemarrhena (Zhimu), Houttuynia (Yuxingcao) and Gypsum (Shigao). 2. Severe cough. *Add:* Tendrilled fritillary bulb (Chuanbeimu) and Trichosanthes skin (Gualoupi). 3. Severe afternoon fever due to *Yin* deficiency. *Add:* Sweet wormwood (Qinghao), Tortoise shell (Biejia) and Fresh rehmannia (Shengdihuang). 4. Severe thirst and irritability. *Add:* Anemarrhena (Zhimu), Glehnia (Shashen) and Trichosanthes root (Tianhuafen).

GEGEN HUANGQIN HUANGLIAN TANG

—Decoction of Pueraria, Scutellaria and Coptis Combination

Pueraria root (Gegen)	15 g
Scutellaria (Huangqin)	9 g
Coptis (Huanglian)	9 g
Licorice (Gancao)	6 g

Method Used: Pueraria root (Gegen) is boiled first, then the other ingredients are boiled together with it by decoction.

Functions: 1. To release the exterior. 2. To clear heat.

Indications: Diarrhea or dysentery caused by dampness and heat.

Manifestations: *Explanations:*

Fever ————————————— Sign of excessive heat.

Diarrhea

Dysentery ————————— Accumulation of dampness and heat in the stomach and intestines impairing the function of the stomach and intestines in transformation and transportation.

Irritability ————————— Mind disturbed by heat and body fluids consumed by heat.

Heat sensation in the chest

Thirst

Red tongue with yellow coating ————————— Signs of excessive heat in the interior.

Rapid pulse

Herbs and Actions:

Pueraria root (Gegen) ————————— To clear heat and release the exterior, ascend *Yang* and stop diarrhea (or dysentery).

Scutellaria (Huangqin) ————————— To clear heat, dry dampness, release toxins and stop dysentery (or diarrhea).

Coptis (Huanglian)

Licorice (Gancao) ————————— To harmonize the actions of the other herbs.

Applications: Acute enteritis and acute dysentery.

Modifications: 1. Dysentery manifested by abdominal pain, bloody stool and tenesmus. *Add:* Pulsatilla root (Baitouweng), Costus root (Muxiang), Bitter orange (Zhiqiao), White peony (Baishao) and Chinese angelica (Danggui). 2. Enteritis manifested by diarrhea. *Add:* Lonicera flower (Jinyinhua), Forsythia (Lianqiao) and Plantain seed (Cheqianzi). 3. Severe abdominal pain. *Add:* Costus root (Muxiang) and White peony (Baishao). 4. Indigestion. *Add:* Hawthorn fruit (Shanzha), Areca seed (Binglang) and Immature bitter orange (Zhishi). 5. Vomiting. *Add:* Pinellia tuber (Banxia) and Fresh ginger (Shengjiang).

SHAOYAO TANG

—Decoction of Peony Combination

White peony (Baishao)	15-20 g
Chinese angelica (Danggui)	9 g
Coptis (Huanglian)	5-9 g
Areca seed (Binglang)	5 g
Costus root (Muxiang)	5 g
Licorice (Gancao)	5 g
Rhubarb (Dahuang)	9 g
Scutellaria (Huangqin)	9 g
Cinnamon twigs (Guizhi)	2-5 g

Method Used: The herbs are cooked by decoction. If the decoction is for dysentery, the herb Rhubarb (Dahuang) should be gradually added during decoction.

Functions: 1. To regulate *Qi* and blood. 2. To clear heat and release toxins.

Indications: Dysentery caused by damp-heat.

Manifestations: *Explanations:*

Abdominal pain

Bloody stool

Tenesmus

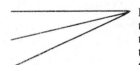

Prolonged accumulation of toxic dampness and heat in the intestines impairing the transportation function of the stomach and intestines.

Hot sensation around the anus

Scanty brown urine

Yellow and sticky tongue coating

Rapid and rolling pulse

Signs of excessive damp-heat in the interior.

Herbs and Actions:

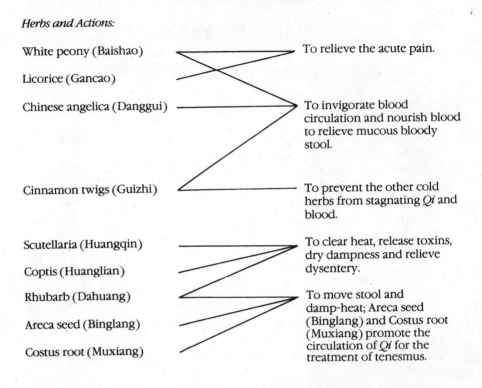

White peony (Baishao)

Licorice (Gancao)

To relieve the acute pain.

Chinese angelica (Danggui)

To invigorate blood circulation and nourish blood to relieve mucous bloody stool.

Cinnamon twigs (Guizhi)

To prevent the other cold herbs from stagnating *Qi* and blood.

Scutellaria (Huangqin)

Coptis (Huanglian)

To clear heat, release toxins, dry dampness and relieve dysentery.

Rhubarb (Dahuang)

Areca seed (Binglang)

Costus root (Muxiang)

To move stool and damp-heat; Areca seed (Binglang) and Costus root (Muxiang) promote the circulation of *Qi* for the treatment of tenesmus.

Applications: Bacterial dysentery and acute enteritis.

Modifications: 1. Severe mucous bloody stool. *Add:* Moutan bark (Mudanpi). 2. Severe tenesmus. *Add:* Bitter orange (Zhiqiao). 3. Indigestion. *Add:* Hawthorn fruit (Shanzha). 4. Severe heat manifestations. *Delete:* Cinnamon twigs (Guizhi).

BAITOUWENG TANG

—Decoction of Chinese Pulsatilla Root Combination

Pulsatilla root (Baitouweng)	15 g
Phellodendron (Huangbai)	12 g
Coptis (Huanglian)	4-6 g
Fraxinus (Qinpi)	12 g

Method Used: The herbs are cooked by decoction.

Functions: 1. To clear heat and release toxins. 2. To cool the blood and relieve dysentery.

Indications: Dysentery due to toxic heat.

Manifestations:	*Explanations:*
Fever	Excessive heat in the interior.
Abdominal pain	Retardation of circulation of *Qi* and blood in the meridians and collaterals.
Bloody stool with pus	Extravasation of bloody by toxic heat.
Tenesmus	*Qi* stagnation and downward attack by pathogenic heat in the intestines.
Burning sensation around the anus	Signs of downward attack by pathogenic heat.
Thirst	Body fluids consumed by heat.
Red tongue with yellow coating	Signs of excessive heat.
Wiry and rapid pulse	

Herbs and Actions:

Pulsatilla root (Baitouweng)	To clear heat, release toxins, cool the blood and relieve dysentery.
Coptis (Huanglian)	To clear heat, dry dampness, release toxins and relieve dysentery.
Phellodendron (Huangbai)	
Fraxinus (Qinpi)	Astringent herb to reduce tenesmus.

Applications: Acute bacillary dysentery and amebic dysentery.

Modifications: 1. Severe abdominal pain and tenesmus. *Add:* Costus root (Muxiang), Bitter orange (Zhiqiao), White peony (Baishao) and Chinese angelica (Danggui). 2. Indigestion. *Add:* Hawthorn fruit (Shanzha), Areca seed (Binglang) and Immature bitter orange (Zhishi). 3. Chills. *Add:* Pueraria root (Gegen) and Lonicera flower (Jinyinhua). 4. Severe fever and heat manifestations. *Add:* Portulaca (Machixian) and Lonicera flower (Jinyinhua). 5. Deficiency of blood. *Add:* Donkey-hide gelatin (Ejiao) and Licorice (Gancao). 6. Pus-like and dark red bloody stool. *Add:* Moutan bark (Mudanpi) and Fresh rehmannia (Shengdihuang). 7. Food-denial dysentery. *Replace:* Phellodendron (Huangbai) with Pilose asiabell root (Dangshen), Ophiopogon root (Maimendong), Caesalpinia (Shilianzi) and Acorus (Changpu).

LIUYI SAN

—Powder of Ingredients Six-to-One in Ratio

Talc (Huashi)	180 g
Licorice (Gancao)	30 g

Method Used: These two can be ground into powder, then mixed with boiled water for oral intake.

Functions: To eliminate dampness, clear heat and relieve summer-heat.

Indications: Damp-heat syndrome caused by invasion of exogenous pathogenic summer-heat and dampness.

Manifestations:

Fever

Thirst

Irritability

Explanations:

Signs of excessive heat and consumption of body fluids.

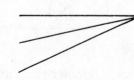

Vomiting

Diarrhea

Dampness and heat remaining in the stomach and intestines and impairing descending function of the stomach, ascending function of the spleen and transportation function of the intestines.

Scanty brown urine

Painful urination

Stranguria by urinary stone

Dampness and heat flowing downward to the urinary bladder and making its *Qi* dysfunction.

Red tongue with yellow coating

Rapid pulse

Signs of excessive dampness and heat.

Herbs and Actions:

Talc (Huashi) ——————————— To clear heat and promote urination.

Licorice (Gancao) ——————————— To prevent Talc (Huashi) from over-promoting urination.

Applications: Acute urinary system infection and acute gastroenteritis.

Modifications: 1. Painful urination and stranguria by urinary stone. *Add:* Lygodium spores (Haijinsha), Lysimachia (Jinqiancao) and Chicken's gizzard skin (Jineijin). 2. Excessive summer-heat manifested by irritability, thirst, and scanty brown urine. *Add:* Watermelon peel (Xiguapi), Luffa sponge (Sigualuo) and Bamboo leaf (Zhuye). 3. Bloody urine, painful urination, frequent urination, and urgent urination. *Add:* Imperata rhizome (Baimaogen), Thistle (Daji), Small thistle (Xiaoji) and Biota tops (Cebaiye). 4. Accompanied manifestations of red eyes, sore throat or ulceration of the mouth and tongue. *Add:* Natural Indigo (Qingdai). This formula is known as Green Jade Powder (Biyusan). 5. Fever and chills. *Add:* Mentha (Bohe). This formula is called Cock-Waking Powder (Jisusan).

QINGSHU YIQI TANG

—Decoction to Clear Summer-Heat and Promote *Qi*

American ginseng (Xiyangshen)	5 g
Dendrobium (Shihu)	15 g
Ophiopogon root (Maimendong)	9 g
Coptis (Huanglian)	3 g
Oryza (Jingmi)	15 g
Bamboo leaf (Zhuye)	6 g
Lotus stem (Hegeng)	15 g
Anemarrhena (Zhimu)	6 g
Licorice (Gancao)	3 g
Watermelon peel (Xiguapi)	30 g

Method Used: The herbs are cooked by decoction.

Functions: 1. To clear summer-heat and promote *Qi*. 2. To replenish *Yin* and promote the production of body fluids.

Indications: Deficiency of both *Qi* and *Yin* due to invasion by summer-heat.

Manifestations:

Fever

Profuse sweating

Irritability

Lassitude

Shortness of breath

Thirst

Rapid and deficient pulse

Red tongue with scanty dry coating

Explanations:

Invasion by exogenous pathogenic summer-heat, making pores open and disturbing the mind.

Signs of deficiency of both *Qi* and *Yin.*

Signs of deficiency of *Qi* and *Yin* caused by heat.

Herbs and Actions:

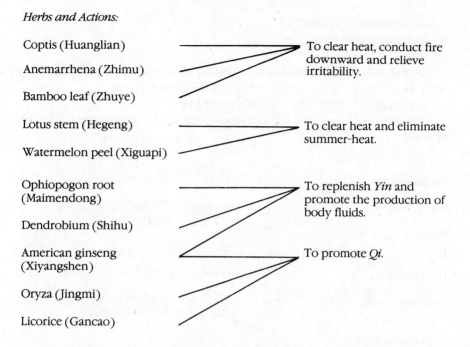

Coptis (Huanglian)

Anemarrhena (Zhimu)

Bamboo leaf (Zhuye)

To clear heat, conduct fire downward and relieve irritability.

Lotus stem (Hegeng)

Watermelon peel (Xiguapi)

To clear heat and eliminate summer-heat.

Ophiopogon root (Maimendong)

Dendrobium (Shihu)

To replenish *Yin* and promote the production of body fluids.

American ginseng (Xiyangshen)

To promote *Qi.*

Oryza (Jingmi)

Licorice (Gancao)

Applications: Summer fever in children and common cold in the summer.

Modifications: Prolonged summer fever in a child. *Replace:* Coptis (Huanglian) with Sweet wormwood (Qinghao), Wolfberry bark (Digupi) and Swallowwort (Baiwei).

QINGHAO BIEJIA TANG

—Decoction of Sweet Wormwood and Tortoise Shell

Sweet wormwood (Qinghao)	6 g
Tortoise shell (Biejia)	15 g
Fresh rehmannia (Shengdihuang)	12 g

Anemarrhena (Zhimu)   6 g
Moutan bark (Mudanpi)   9 g

Method Used: The herbs and substances are cooked by decoction with five cups of water until two cups of liquid remain.

Functions: To replenish *Yin* and dispel heat.

Indications: Deficiency of *Yin* and heat in the late stage of febrile diseases.

Manifestations:

Fever at night

No sweating when fever is gone

Emaciation

Red tongue with scanty coating

Rapid pulse

Explanations:

Deficiency of *Yin* and existence of heat.

Deficiency of *Yin* and blood.

Signs of deficiency of *Yin* and internal heat.

Herbs and Actions:

Sweet Wormwood (Qinghao)

Moutan bark (Mudanpi)

Tortoise shell (Biejia)

Anemarrhena (Zhimu)

Fresh rehmannia (Shengdihuang)

Fragrant and cold herbs to clear heat and cool the blood.

To replenish *Yin* and dispel heat.

Applications: Summer fever in children and low grade fever due to chronic infection.

Modifications: 1. Severe *Yin* deficiency. *Add:* Ophiopogon root (Maimendong), White peony (Baishao) and Scrophularia (Xuanshen). 2. Excessive heat. *Add:* Stellaria (Yinchaihu), Eclipta (Hanliancao) and Swallowwort (Baiwei).

QINGGU SAN

—Powder to Clear Heat in the Bones

Stellaria (Yinchaihu)	5 g
Wolfberry bark (Digupi)	3 g
Picrorrhiza (Huhuanglian)	3 g
Sweet wormwood (Qinghao)	3 g
Large-leaf gentiana (Qinjiao)	3 g
Anemarrhena (Zhimu)	3 g
Tortoise shell (Biejia)	3 g
Licorice (Gancao)	2 g

Method Used: The herbs and substances are cooked by decoction.
Functions: 1. To clear heat caused by deficiency of *Yin*. 2. To relieve afternoon fever and bone-steaming sensation.
Indications: *Yin* deficiency and internal heat.

Manifestations:

Explanations:

Fever at night

Afternoon fever

Night sweating

Deficient *Yin* depressed by *Yang* which steams body fluids.

Feverish sensation on the palms, soles and in the chest

Yin deficiency and internal heat.

Emaciation

Yin and body fluids all consumed.

Red lips

Malar flushed

Flaring up of fire caused by *Yin* deficiency.

Red tongue with little coating

Threativy and rapid pulse.

Signs of internal heat by *Yin* deficiency.

91

Herbs and Actions:

Anemarrhena (Zhimu) ——————— To replenish *Yin* and clear
                                                            heat.
Tortoise shell (Biejia)

Picrorrhiza (Huhuanglian) ——————— To clear heat by *Yin*
                                                                deficiency and relieve
Wolfberry bark (Digupi)   afternoon fever with
                                                                sweating.

Sweet wormwood (Qinghao) ——————— To clear heat by *Yin*
                                                                      deficiency but relieve
Large-leaf gentiana (Qinjiao)   afternoon fever without
                                                                      sweating.

Licorice (Gancao)   ——————— To harmonize the actions of
                                                            the other herbs and prevent
                                                            them from injuring the
                                                            stomach.

Applications: Active tuberculosis.

Modifications: 1. Severe *Yin* deficiency. *Add:* Fresh rehmannia (Sheng-dihuang), White peony (Baishao) and Chinese angelica (Danggui). 2. *Qi* deficiency. *Add:* Astragalus (Huangqi). 3. Diarrhea and poor appetite. *Replace:* Anemarrhena (Zhimu) and Picrorrhiza (Huhuanglian) with Dolichos seed (Biandou) and Dioscorea (Shanyao). 4. Cough or cough with blood. *Add:* Donkey-hide gelatin (Ejiao), Ophiopogon root (Mai-mendong) and Schisandra fruit (Wuweizi). 5. Profuse sweating. *Add:* Astragalus (Huangqi) and Oyster shell (Shengmuli).

DANGGUI LIUHUANG TANG

—Decoction of Chinese Angelica and
Six Yellow Ingredients

Chinese angelica (Danggui)   9 g
Fresh rehmannia (Shengdihuang)   9 g

Coptis (Huanglian)	9 g
Prepared rehmannia (Shudihuang)	9 g
Scutellaria (Huangqin)	9 g
Phellodendron (Huangbai)	9 g
Astragalus (Huangqi)	18 g

Method Used: The herbs are cooked with water by decoction.

Functions: 1. To replenish *Yin* and reduce fire. 2. To consolidate the exterior and stop sweating.

Indications: Night sweating by *Yin* deficiency with excessive fire and impairment of the pores' function.

Manifestations: *Explanations:*

Night sweating ——————————— *Yin* deficiency and excessive fire which impair the function of pores, leading to body fluids flowing out.

Red face

Irritability —————————— Flaring up of fire which disturbs the mind.

Dry mouth and lips

Constipation —————————— Deficiency of body fluids.

Yellow urine

Red tongue proper —————————— Signs of *Yin* deficiency with fire in the interior.

Rapid pulse

Herbs and Actions:

Chinese angelica (Danggui)

Fresh rehmannia
(Shengdihuang) —————————— To replenish *Yin*, nourish blood and clear heat.

Prepared rehmannia
(Shudihuang)

93

Scutellaria (Huangqin)

Phellodendron (Huangbai)

Coptis (Huanglian)

To clear heat, reduce fire and relieve irritability.

Astragalus (Huangqi) ———————————— To tonify *Qi* and consolidate the exterior.

Applications: Night sweating.

Modifications: Manifestations of afternoon fever, red tongue with little coating, thready and rapid pulse. *Replace:* Phellodendron (Huangbai), Scutellaria (Huangqin) and Coptis (Huanglian) with Anemarrhena (Zhimu) and Tortoise plastron (Guiban).

Cautions: The formula is contraindicated for a person with weakness of the spleen and stomach, poor appetite and loose stool.

V. Formulas to Dispel Cold

Formulas composed chiefly of warm or hot natured herbs intended to warm *Yang*, dispel cold and treat interior cold syndromes are called dispelling cold formulas. They can be divided into three categories:

1. Formulas for warming the spleen and stomach and dispelling cold. They warm the spleen and stomach and are used to treat syndromes caused by deficiency and coldness in the middle *jiao*.

2. Formulas for restoring *Yang* from collapse. They recuperate depleted *Yang* and rescue the patient from collapse and are used to treat syndromes caused by declined *Yang* with excessive *Yin* or sudden collapse of *Yang*.

3. Formulas for warming meridians and dispelling cold. They warm meridians and are used to treat syndromes caused by coldness in the meridians.

LIZHONG WAN

—Pills to Regulate the Middle *Jiao* (Spleen and Stomach)

Ginseng (Renshen)	6 g
Licorice (Gancao)	6 g

Dried ginger (Ganjiang)   5 g
White atractylodes (Baizhu)   9 g

Method Used: The herbs are ground into powder, and then mixed with honey to make pills.

Functions: 1. To warm the middle *jiao* (spleen and stomach) and dispel cold. 2. To tonify *Qi* and strengthen the spleen.

Indications: Weakness and coldness of the spleen and stomach, such as: (a) stomach and intestine disorders; (b) loss of blood due to spleen *Yang* deficiency; (c) infantile convulsions; (d) obstruction in the chest.

Manifestations: *Explanations:*

1. Stomach and intestine
   disorders:

Nausea   Weakness and coldness of the
                                                spleen and stomach failing its
Vomiting   functions of transformation
                                                and transportation, ascending
Diarrhea   and descending.

No thirst ————————————————— Existence of dampness.

Abdominal distention ————————— *Qi* stagnation by cold.

Abdominal pain

Poor appetite ————————————— Weakness of the spleen and
                                                stomach.

Cold limbs ——————————————— Deficiency of spleen *Yang*
                                                which cannot warm up the
                                                limbs.

2. Lose of blood due to spleen
   Yang deficiency:

Bloody stool   *Yang* deficiency of the spleen
                                                making the organ fail its
Uterine bleeding   function of controlling blood.

Profuse menstrual flow

3. Infantile convulsions:

Convulsions of the four limbs ———————————— Weakness of the spleen
failing to dominate the
muscles of the four limbs.

4. Obstruction in the chest:

Chest pain ————————————————— Production of phlegm due to
spleen blocking in the chest.
Stifling sensation in the chest

Pale tongue ————————————————— Signs of *Yang* deficiency and
existence of phlegm and
White and sticky or white
dampness in the interior.
and watery coating

Deep, thready and forceless
or slow and tardy pulse

Herbs and Actions:

Ginseng (Renshen) ———————————— To tonify *Qi* in the spleen and
stomach and strengthen the
White atractylodes (Baizhu)
spleen to resolve dampness.

Licorice (Gancao)

Dried ginger (Ganjiang) ————————— To warm the middle *jiao* and
dispel coldness.

Applications: Indigestion, chronic diarrhea, functional uterine bleeding, bloody stool due to gastroduodenal ulcer and angina pectoris.

Modifications: 1. Severe vomiting. *Replace:* White atractylodes (Baizhu) with Fresh ginger (Shengjiang) and Cloves (Dingxiang). 2. Severe abdominal pain and distention. *Add:* Aconite (Fuzi). 3. Severe diarrhea. *Add:* Dioscorea (Shanyao), Dolichos seed (Biandou) and Poria (Fuling). 4. Loss of blood due to *Yang* deficiency. *Add:* Donkey-hide gelatin (Ejiao), Chinese mugwort leaf (Aiye) and Antler gelatin (Lujiaojiao). 5. **Pain in the chest. Add: Red sage root (Danshen), Trichosanthes (Gualou), Curcuma root (Yujin) and Bitter orange (Zhiqiao). 6. Infantile convulsions. Add: Uncaria stem (Gouteng), White stiff silkworm (Jiangcan) and Gastrodia tuber (Tianma). 7. Leukorrhagia** due to flowing

97

downward of the dampness produced by weakness and coldness of the spleen. *Add:* Dodder seed (Tusizi), Deglued antler powder (Lujiaoshuang), Dioscorea (Shanyao), Poria (Fuling), Baked coix seed (Chaoyiren) and Oyster shell (Shengmuli).

WUZHUYU TANG

—Decoction of Evodia Fruit Combination

Evodia fruit (Wuzhuyu)	3 g
Jujube (Dazao)	4 pcs
Ginseng (Renshen)	6 g
Fresh ginger (Shengjiang)	18 g

Method Used: The herbs are cooked by decoction.

Functions: 1. To warm and tonify the spleen and stomach. 2. To conduct perversion of *Qi* downward and stop vomiting.

Indications: Vomiting due to weakness and coldness in the spleen and stomach and perversion of *Qi*.

Manifestations:

Explanations:

1. Vomiting immediately after intake of food

Stifling sensation and fullness in the epigastric region

Epigastric pain

Acid regurgitation

Weakness and coldness of the spleen and stomach leading to upward perversion of the stomach *Qi*, dysfunction of the spleen in transformation and transportation, retention of the turbid phlegm and stagnation of *Qi*.

2. Retching

Vomiting with saliva

Upward perversion of the stomach *Qi* and harmful water.

Vertex headache

Upward attack of the liver *Qi* affected by weakness and coldness of the spleen and stomach.

3. Vomiting ⟶ Weakness and coldness of the spleen and stomach leading

Diarrhea to internal retention of harmful water and dampness and dysfunction of the spleen and stomach in ascending and descending.

Cold limbs ⟶ Excess cold leading to *Yang* deficiency which cannot warm the limbs.

Irritability ⟶ Excess cold leading to a struggle between *Yin* and *Yang*.

Pale tongue with white and watery coating ⟶ Cold, retention of dampness and turbid phlegm fluid.

Slow pulse

Herbs and Actions:

Evodia fruit (Wuzhuyu) ⟶ To ease the liver, check the acid and stop pain.

Fresh ginger (Shengjiang) ⟶ To dispel cold, conduct perversion of *Qi* downward and relieve vomiting.

Ginseng (Renshen) ⟶ To tonify *Qi* of the spleen and stomach.

Jujube (Dazao)

Applications: Acute and chronic gastritis, neurotic headache, Meniere's syndrome and migraine.

Modifications: 1. Severe headache. *Add:* Ligusticum (Chuanxiong) and Sichuan chinaberry (Chuanlianzi). 2. Severe vomiting. *Add:* Pinellia tuber (Banxia), Amomum (Sharen) and Citrus peel (Jupi).

Cautions: This decoction may induce further vomiting. It should be taken cold and more frequently.

XIAO JIANZHONG TANG

—Minor Decoction to Restore the Normal Function of the Middle *Jiao*

White peony (Baishao)	18 g
Cinnamon twigs (Guizhi)	9 g
Licorice (Gancao)	6 g
Fresh ginger (Shengjiang)	10 g
Jujube (Dazao)	12 pcs
Maltose (Yitang)	30 g

Method Used: The five herbs are first cooked by decoction, then Maltose (Yitang) is added.

Functions: 1. To warm and tonify the middle *jiao* (spleen and stomach). 2. To dispel cold and stop pain.

Indications: Abdominal pain due to weakness and coldness in the spleen and stomach.

Manifestations:

Explanations:

Paroxysmal pain in the epigastrium (relieved by warmth and pressure)

Weakness and coldness in the spleen and stomach.

Pathogenic cold blocking the meridians and collaterals and giving rise to pain.

Pale tongue proper with thin and white coating

Signs of deficiency and cold.

Thready and weak pulse

Herbs and Actions:

Cinnamon twigs (Guizhi)

To warm the spleen and stomach, dispel cold and promote the circulation of meridians and collaterals.

100

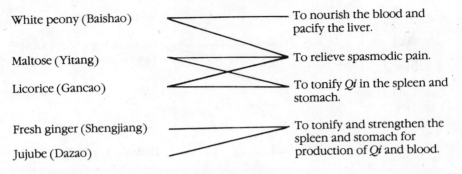

White peony (Baishao) — To nourish the blood and pacify the liver.

Maltose (Yitang) — To relieve spasmodic pain.

Licorice (Gancao) — To tonify *Qi* in the spleen and stomach.

Fresh ginger (Shengjiang) — To tonify and strengthen the spleen and stomach for

Jujube (Dazao) — production of *Qi* and blood.

Applications: Gastric and duodenal ulcers.

Modifications: 1. Severe blood deficiency. *Add:* Chinese angelica (Danggui). The formula is called Danggui Jianzhong Tang. 2. Severe *Qi* deficiency. *Add:* Astragalus (Huangqi). The formula is called Huangqi Jianzhong Tang. 3. This decoction can also be used to treat blood deficiency, which cannot nourish the heart, manifesting by palpitation, insomnia, pale complexion, pale tongue with white coating, thready and weak pulse.

SINI TANG

—Decoction to Treat Cold Limbs

Aconite (Fuzi)	5-10 g
Dried ginger (Ganjiang)	6-9 g
Licorice (Gancao)	6 g

Method Used: First, Aconite (Fuzi) should be cooked for an hour. Then the other two herbs are added to the decoction for cooking.

Functions: To restore the *Yang* after collapse.

Indications: Syndrome of excessive *Yin* and declined *Yang*.

Manifestations: — *Explanations:*

1. Cold limbs

Aversion to cold

Curled up sleep

Yang deficiency failing to warm up the limbs.

Fatigued and sleepy ——————————— Signs of *Yang* deficiency.

Vomiting ————————————— Manifestations of declined
Yang of the spleen.
Diarrhea

Abdominal pain

Indigestion

No thirst ——————————— Deficiency of *Yang* causing
dampness.

Pale tongue with white ——————————— Signs of excess *Yin* and
coating declined *Yang*.

Thready and forceless pulse

2. Profuse sweating ——————————— Excessive *Yin* and collapsed
Yang.

Cold limbs ——————————— *Yang* deficiency of the heart
failing to house the mind and
Listlessness general *Yang* deficiency
failing to warm up the limbs.
Coma

Pale complexion ——————————— Declined *Yang* failing to push
the circulation of *Qi* and
Cyanosis on the lips and nails blood.

Weak, thready and fading
pulse

Pale tongue and white ——————————— Signs of excessive *Yin* and
coating declined *Yang*.

Herbs and Actions:

Aconite (Fuzi) ——————————— To restore *Yang* and dispel
cold.

Dried ginger (Ganjiang) ——————————— To warm the spleen and
stomach and dispel cold.

Licorice (Gancao) ——————————— To harmonize the actions of
the other herbs and promote
Qi circulation.

Applications: Coma.
Modifications: Severe coma. *Add:* Ginseng (Renshen).

SHEN FU TANG

—Decoction of Ginseng and Aconite

Ginseng (Renshen)	9 g
Aconite (Fuzi)	6 g

Method Used: The two herbs are cooked by decoction.
Functions: To restore the *Yang Qi.*
Indications: Yang Qi collapsing syndrome due to the source *Qi* being greatly damaged.

Manifestations: *Explanations:*

Profuse sweating ———————— Damage of the source *Qi* impairing the defensive *Qi,* leading to dysfunction of pores in opening and closing.

Cold limbs ———————— Deficiency of *Yang Qi* failing to warm up the limbs.

Feeble breath ———————— *Qi* deficiency.

Weak, fading pulse ———————— Signs of deficiency of *Yang Qi* which fails in pushing circulation of the blood.

Herbs and Actions:

Ginseng (Renshen) ———————— To tonify source *Qi,* replenish *Yin* and promote production of body fluids.

Aconite (Fuzi) ———————— To prevent collapse and stop sweating.

To warm and strengthen the source *Yang.*

103

Applications: Cardiac failure and coma.

Modifications: Profuse sweating and thirst. *Add:* Ophiopogon root (Maimendong) and Schisandra fruit (Wuweizi).

ZHENWU TANG

—Decoction of Aconite, White Atractytodes and Poria Combination

Poria (Fuling)	9 g
White peony (Baishao)	9 g
White atractylodes (Baizhu)	6 g
Aconite (Fuzi)	9 g
Fresh ginger (Shengjiang)	9 g

Method Used: The herbs are cooked with water by decoction.

Functions: To warm *Yang* and promote water-metabolism.

Indications: Retention of water due to deficiency of *Yang* of the spleen and kidneys.

Manifestations:

Dysuria

Edema in the limbs and body

Heavy sensation in the four limbs

Severe chills

Abdominal pain

Loose stool

No thirst

Explanations:

Deficiency of *Yang* of the spleen and kidney failing to control the water-metabolism.

Yang deficiency.

Deficiency of *Yang* of the spleen and kidney giving rise to coldness and retention of dampness.

104

Pale tongue with white coating ——————————→ Signs of *Yang* deficiency.

Deep and forceless pulse

Palpitation ——————————→ The heart and lungs attacked by the upward flow of harmful water.

Shortness of breath

Dizziness —————————— Depressed, clean *Yang* failing to ascend to the head to nourish the mind because of retention of water.

Lassitude —————————— Deficiency of *Yang Qi*.

Herbs and Actions:

Aconite (Fuzi) ——————————→ To warm *Yang*, dispel cold and promote water-metabolism.

Fresh ginger (Shengjiang)

White atractylodes (Baizhu) ——————————→ To promote *Qi* circulation, strengthen the spleen, promote urination and reduce edema.

Poria (Fuling)

White peony (Baishao) —————————— To replenish *Yin* and blood, stop pain and prevent the actions of the other herbs from consuming *Yin* and blood.

Applications: Cardiac failure, hypothyroidism, chronic diarrhea, trophedema, Sheehan's disease and Addison's disease.

Modifications: Severe edema. *Add:* Cinnamon twigs (Guizhi), Polyporus (Zhuling) and Alisma (Zexie).

DANGGUI SINI TANG

—Decoction of Chinese Angelica Combination to Treat Cold Limbs

Chinese angelica (Danggui)	12 g
Cinnamon twigs (Guizhi)	9 g
White peony (Baishao)	9 g
Asarum (Xixin)	1.5 g
Licorice (Gancao)	5 g
Ricepaper pith (Tongcao)	3 g
Jujube (Dazao)	8 pcs

Method Used: The herbs are cooked with water by decoction.

Functions: 1. To warm meridians and dispel cold. 2. To nourish the blood.

Indications: Cold hands and feet caused by deficiency of blood and cold.

Manifestations:

Explanations:

Cold limbs

Cold pain

Deficiency of blood unable to warm the limbs and invasion of exogenous pathogenic cold retarding the circulation of the blood and blocking the blood vessels.

Pale tongue with white coating

Deep, thready and fading pulse

Signs of blood deficiency with cold.

Herbs and Actions:

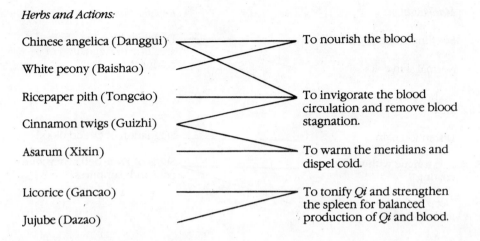

Chinese angelica (Danggui)

White peony (Baishao)

To nourish the blood.

Ricepaper pith (Tongcao)

Cinnamon twigs (Guizhi)

To invigorate the blood circulation and remove blood stagnation.

Asarum (Xixin)

To warm the meridians and dispel cold.

Licorice (Gancao)

Jujube (Dazao)

To tonify *Qi* and strengthen the spleen for balanced production of *Qi* and blood.

Applications: Thromboangiitis, athetosis, frostbite, dysmenorrhea and chronic rheumatoid arthritis.

Modifications: Dysmenorrhea. *Add:* Lindera root (Wuyao) and Fennel fruit (Xiaohuixiang).

YANGHE TANG
—Decoction of Prepared Rehmannia, Cinnamon Bark and Ephedra Combination

Prepared rehmannia (Shudihuang)	30 g
Cinnamon bark (Rougui)	3 g
Ephedra (Mahuang)	2 g
Antler gelatin (Lujiaojiao)	9 g
Brassia seed (Baijiezi)	6 g
Baked ginger (Paojiang)	2 g
Licorice (Gancao)	3 g

Method Used: The herbs are cooked with water by decoction.

Functions: 1. To warm the *Yang* and tonify blood. 2. To dispel cold and remove stagnation.

Indications: Deep-rooted boils caused by blood deficiency and cold.

Manifestations:

Swelling without pus ⟶

Normal skin color ⟶

No hot feeling in affected area ⟶

Explanations:

Deficient blood in affected area due to stagnation of coldness.

Distention pain ⟶ Stagnation of *Qi* and blood.

Pale tongue with white coating ⟶

Deep and thready or deep and slow pulse ⟶

Signs of *Yang* deficiency with cold and dampness.

Herbs and Actions:

Prepared rehmannia (Shudihuang) ⟶

Antler gelatin (Lujiaojiao) ⟶

To tonify blood and essence and encourage the formation of pus to eliminate toxins.

Cinnamon bark (Rougui) ⟶

Baked ginger (Paojiang) ⟶

To dispel cold, remove stagnation and speed up the formation of pus.

Ephedra (Mahuang) ⟶

Brassia seed (Baijiezi) ⟶

To resolve phlegm, remove stagnation and relieve nodules and boils.

Licorice (Gancao) ⟶ To harmonize the actions of the other herbs and release toxins.

Applications: Thromboangiitis, rheumatoid arthritis, boils and bone tuberculosis.

Modifications: 1. *Qi* deficiency. *Add:* Ginseng (Renshen) and Astragalus (Huangqi). 2. Excess cold. *Add:* Aconite (Fuzi).

Cautions: The formula is contraindicated in a person with *Yin* deficiency with heat manifestations, boils with ulcers and breast cancer.

VI. Tonic Formulas

Formulas that nourish and strengthen inadequacy of *Qi*, blood, *Yin* and *Yang* of the body and treat deficient syndromes are called tonic formulas. They can be divided into four categories:

1. *Qi* tonic formulas. They tonify *Qi* and are used to treat *Qi* deficient syndromes.

2. Blood tonic formulas. They tonify blood and are used to treat syndromes of blood deficiency.

3. *Yin* tonic formulas. They tonify *Yin* and are used to treat syndromes caused by *Yin* deficiency.

4. *Yang* tonic formulas. They tonify *Yang* and are used to treat *Yang* deficiency syndromes.

Cautions: Large dosages of tonic formulas may injure the stomach. They should be used with caution with a person who has excess internal pathogenic factors.

SIJUNZI TANG

—The Four Noble Ingredients Decoction

Ginseng (Renshen)	10 g
Poria (Fuling)	9 g
White atractylodes (Baizhu)	9 g
Licorice (Gancao)	6 g

Method Used: The herbs are ground into powder and then cooked with water by decoction.

Functions: To tonify *Qi* and strengthen the spleen.

Indications: Deficiency of *Qi* in the spleen and stomach in which transformation and transportation are weak.

Manifestations: *Explanations:*

Pale face ——————————————— Manifestations of *Qi* deficiency.

Weak voice

Weakness of four limbs ———————— *Qi* deficiency in the spleen which fails to control the muscles of the limbs.

Loss of appetite ———————————— Weakness of the spleen and stomach which fail in transformation and transportation, giving rise to dampness and causing impairment of the functions of ascending and descending.

Borborygmus

Diarrhea or loose stool

Nausea

Vomiting

Pale tongue with thin and ———————— Signs of *Qi* deficiency.
white coating

Deficient and forceless pulse

Herbs and Actions:

Ginseng (Renshen) ——————————— To tonify *Qi* in the spleen and stomach and strengthen the spleen.

White atractylodes (Baizhu)

Poria (Fuling) ——————————————— To eliminate dampness, strengthen the spleen and stop diarrhea.

Licorice (Gancao) ——————————— To harmonize actions of the other herbs.

Applications: Chronic gastritis, gastric and duodenal ulcers and stomach and intestine disorders.

Modifications: 1. *Qi* stagnation manifested by stifling sensation and fullness in the chest and epigastric region. *Add:* Citrus peel (Jupi). This formula is known as Wuwei Yigong San. 2. Cough with profuse, white, diluted sputum. *Add:* Citrus peel (Jupi), Pinellia tuber (Banxia), Fresh ginger (Shengjiang) and Jujube (Dazao). This formula is called Liujunzi Tang. 3. Distention and fullness in the epigastric and abdominal regions, vomiting, diarrhea and abdominal pain. *Add:* Costus root (Muxiang), Amomum (Sharen), Citrus peel (Jupi), Pinellia tuber (Banxia) and Fresh ginger (Shengjiang). This formula is called Xiangsha Liujunzi Tang. 4. Deficiency of *Qi* and blood. *Add:* Chinese angelica (Danggui), White peony (Baishao), Prepared rehmannia (Shudihuang) and Ligusticum (Chuanxiong). This formula is called Bazhen Tang. 5. Weakness of the spleen and excessive dampness manifested by vomiting, diarrhea and poor appetite. *Add:* Astragalus (Huangqi) and Dolichos seed (Biandou).

BUZHONG YIQI TANG

—Decoction to Reinforce the Middle *Jiao* and Tonify *Qi*

Astragalus (Huangqi)	15-20 g
Licorice (Gancao)	5 g
Ginseng (Renshen)	10 g
Chinese angelica (Danggui)	10 g
Citrus peel (Jupi)	6 g
Cimicifuga (Shengma)	3 g
Bupleurum (Chaihu)	3 g
White atractylodes (Baizhu)	10 g

Method Used: The herbs are cooked with water by decoction.

Functions: 1. To reinforce the middle *jiao* and tonify *Qi*. 2. To uplift the *Yang* and relieve phosis.

Indications: Syndrome of deficiency of *Qi* in the spleen and stomach and prolapse of viscera due to sinking of *Yang Qi*.

Manifestations:

Explanations:

1. Deficiency of *Qi* in the
   spleen and stomach:

Pale complexion ——————————— *Qi* deficiency.

Laziness in speech

Fatigue ——————————— Weakness of the spleen
which cannot control
muscles.

Poor appetite ——————————— Impairment of
transformation and
Loose stool ——————————— transportation of the spleen
leading to existence of
dampness.

Fever ——————————— *Yang Qi* sinking into the *Yin*
portion due to deficiency of
the spleen.

Spontaneous sweating ——————————— Weakness of the spleen
causing *Qi* deficiency and
disturbing the pores' ability
to open and close.

Pale tongue with thin and ——————————— Signs of *Qi* deficiency.
white coating

Big and deficient pulse

2. Sinking of *Yang Qi:*

Prolapse of rectum ——————————— *Qi* deficiency of the spleen
and stomach making *Qi* sink
Prolapse of uterus and fail in uplifting.

Gastroptosis

Prolonged diarrhea

Chronic dysentery

Pale tongue with thin and ——————————— Signs of *Qi* deficiency.
white coating

Big and deficient pulse

Herbs and Actions:

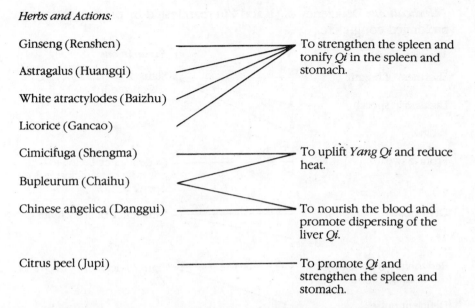

Ginseng (Renshen)

Astragalus (Huangqi)

White atractylodes (Baizhu)

Licorice (Gancao)

To strengthen the spleen and tonify *Qi* in the spleen and stomach.

Cimicifuga (Shengma)

Bupleurum (Chaihu)

To uplift *Yang Qi* and reduce heat.

Chinese angelica (Danggui)

To nourish the blood and promote dispersing of the liver *Qi*.

Citrus peel (Jupi)

To promote *Qi* and strengthen the spleen and stomach.

Applications: Prolapse of viscera, anemia, chronic gastritis, chronic hepatitis, chronic enteritis and common cold with weak constitution.

Modifications: Collapse of viscera due to sinking of *Qi* in the middle *jiao*. *Add:* Bitter orange (Zhiqiao) and Astragalus (Huangqi) in large dosage.

SHENGMAI SAN

—Powder to Activate Vitality

Ginseng (Renshen)	10 g
Schisandra fruit (Wuweizi)	6 g
Ophiopogon root (Maimendong)	15 g

Method Used: The herbs are cooked with water three times by decoction.

Functions: 1. To tonify *Qi* and promote the production of body fluids. 2. To astringe *Yin* and stop sweating.

Indications: Deficiency of *Qi* and *Yin* manifested by profuse sweating, prolonged cough, etc.

Manifestations:	*Explanations:*
Shortness of breath	Signs of *Qi* deficiency in the spleen and lungs.
Laziness in speech	
Fatigue	
Profuse sweating	*Qi* deficiency failing to control pores in closing and opening.
Dry throat	Deficiency of body fluids.
Thirst	
Red tongue with scanty and dry coating	Signs of deficiency of *Qi* and *Yin*.
Deficient pulse	
Dry cough with sputum	Deficiency of body fluids.
Dry throat	
Dry tongue	
Shortness of breath	*Qi* deficiency and dysfunction of pores in opening and closing.
Lassitude	
Spontaneous sweating	
Red tongue with dry and little coating	Signs of deficiency of *Qi* and *Yin*.
Deficient pulse	

Herbs and Actions:

Ginseng (Renshen)	To tonify *Qi* and promote the production of body fluids.
Ophiopogon root (Maimendong)	To replenish *Yin*, moisten dryness and clear heat.

| Schisandra fruit (Wuweizi) | To astringe *Yin Qi* and stop sweating and cough. |

Applications: Coma, cardiac failure, neurasthenia and arrhythmia.

Modifications: 1. Severe damage of *Yin* and body fluids manifested by mild heat. *Add:* Scrophularia (Xuanshen) and Fresh rehmannia (Shengdihuang). 2. Prolonged cough. *Add:* Stemona root (Baibu). 3. Palpitation and insomnia. *Add:* Wild jujube seed (Suanzaoren), Dragon's bone (Longgu) and Oyster shell (Shengmuli).

Cautions: The formula points to deficiency of *Qi* and *Yin* caused by summer-heat attack, but it does not have the ability to clear heat and dispel summer-heat. So, if a fever caused by summer-heat remains, this formula cannot be used.

SIWU TANG

—The Four Ingredients Decoction

Prepared rehmannia (Shudihuang)	12 g
Chinese angelica (Danggui)	10 g
Ligusticum (Chuanxiong)	8 g
White peony (Baishao)	12 g

Method Used: The herbs are cooked with water three times by decoction. The decoction is taken before meals.

Functions: To nourish and invigorate blood.

Indications: Blood deficiency and stagnant blood.

Manifestations:

Dizziness

Vertigo

Tinnitus

Palpitation

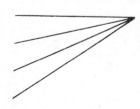

Explanations:

Blood deficiency failing to nourish the head, eyes and mind.

Irregular menstruation

Abdominal pain

Blood deficiency and stagnant blood, which retard the circulation of blood and fail to nourish the Chong and Ren meridians.

Pale lips and nails

Pale tongue proper

Wiry and thready or thready and choppy pulse

Signs of blood deficiency.

Herbs and Actions:

Chinese angelica (Danggui)

Ligusticum (Chuanxiong)

Prepared rehmannia (Shudihuang)

White peony (Baishao)

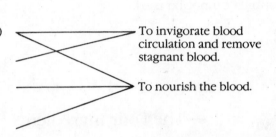

To invigorate blood circulation and remove stagnant blood.

To nourish the blood.

Applications: Irregular menstruation and anemia.

Modifications: 1. Severe stagnant blood manifested by abdominal pain. *Add:* Peach seed (Taoren) and Carthamus (Honghua). 2. *Qi* stagnation manifested by abdominal distention. *Add:* Cyperus tuber (Xiangfu) and Lindera root (Wuyao). 3. *Qi* deficiency manifested by shortness of breath and lassitude. *Add:* Ginseng (Renshen) and Astragalus (Huangqi). 4. Uterine bleeding due to threatened abortion. *Add:* Donkey-hide gelatin (Ejiao) and Chinese mugwort leaf (Aiye). 5. More cold manifestations. *Add:* Cinnamon bark (Rougui) and Baked ginger (Paojiang). More heat manifestations. *Add:* Scutellaria (Huangqin) and Capejasmine fruit (Zhizi). 6. Severe blood deficiency. *Add:* Fleece flower root (Heshouwu), Lycium fruit (Gouqizi) and Dodder seed (Tusizi).

116

DANGGUI BUXUE TANG

—Decoction with Chinese Angelica Combination to Tonify Blood

Astragalus (Huangqi)	30 g
Chinese angelica (Danggui)	6 g

Method Used: The herbs are cooked with water three time by decoction. The decoction is taken before meals.

Functions: To tonify *Qi* and promote the production of blood.

Indications: Blood deficiency and floating of *Yang* due to fatigue and deficiency of source *Qi*.

Manifestations:

Explanations:

Hot sensation of the body

Red face

Thirst

Want to drink

Deficiency of *Yin* blood, which cannot control *Yang*, leading to upward flowing of *Yang Qi*.

Surging, big and deficient pulse — Sign of blood deficiency and flowing of *Yang*.

Anemia and heat manifestation in post-partus or menstruation period — Blood deficiency leading to floating of *Yang*.

Headache — Blood deficiency which cannot nourish the head.

Purulent abscesses — *Qi* and blood deficiency failing to promote the production of new muscles.

Herbs and Actions:

Chinese angelica (Danggui) — To nourish blood and control the *Yang*.

117

Astragalus (Huangqi) ——————————— To tonify *Qi* and nourish blood.

Applications: Anemia, uterine bleeding, post-partus bleeding and fever and purulent abscesses.

Cautions: 1. Heat manifestation here is due to the deficiency of blood leading to the failure of *Yang*, so heat here should not be regarded as a sign of common fever. Cold or cool herbs should be avoided as such formulas may worsen the disease. 2. This formula is contraindicated for a person with *Yin* deficiency manifested by afternoon fever.

GUIPI TANG

—Decoction to Strengthen the Spleen and Heart

White atractylodes (Baizhu)	30 g
Poria (Fuling)	30 g
Astragalus (Huangqi)	30 g
Longan aril (Longyanrou)	30 g
Wild jujube seed (Suanzaoren)	30 g
Ginseng (Renshen)	15 g
Costus root (Muxiang)	15 g
Licorice (Gancao)	8 g
Chinese angelica (Danggui)	3 g
Polygala root (Yuanzhi)	3 g

Method Used: Once the herbs are mixed, six grams of Fresh ginger (Shengjiang) and three pieces of Jujube (Dazao) are added to the herbs which are then cooked with water by decoction.

Functions: 1. To tonify *Qi* and blood. 2. To strengthen the spleen and heart.

Indications: Spleen and heart deficiency or *Qi* and blood deficiency due to fatigue or over-thinking.

118

TONIC FORMULAS

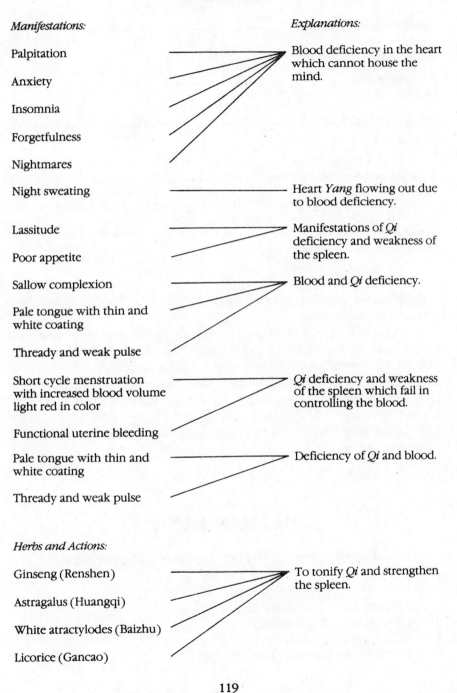

Manifestations:

Palpitation

Anxiety

Insomnia

Forgetfulness

Nightmares

Night sweating

Lassitude

Poor appetite

Sallow complexion

Pale tongue with thin and white coating

Thready and weak pulse

Short cycle menstruation with increased blood volume light red in color

Functional uterine bleeding

Pale tongue with thin and white coating

Thready and weak pulse

Herbs and Actions:

Ginseng (Renshen)

Astragalus (Huangqi)

White atractylodes (Baizhu)

Licorice (Gancao)

Explanations:

Blood deficiency in the heart which cannot house the mind.

Heart *Yang* flowing out due to blood deficiency.

Manifestations of *Qi* deficiency and weakness of the spleen.

Blood and *Qi* deficiency.

Qi deficiency and weakness of the spleen which fail in controlling the blood.

Deficiency of *Qi* and blood.

To tonify *Qi* and strengthen the spleen.

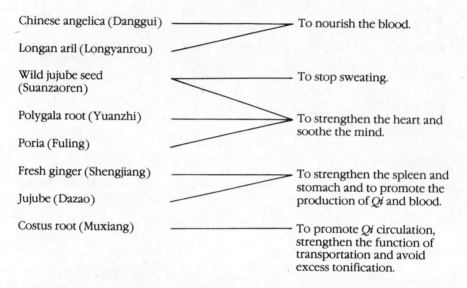

Chinese angelica (Danggui) —————— To nourish the blood.

Longan aril (Longyanrou)

Wild jujube seed —————— To stop sweating.
(Suanzaoren)

Polygala root (Yuanzhi) —————— To strengthen the heart and
soothe the mind.
Poria (Fuling)

Fresh ginger (Shengjiang) —————— To strengthen the spleen and
stomach and to promote the
Jujube (Dazao) production of *Qi* and blood.

Costus root (Muxiang) —————— To promote *Qi* circulation,
strengthen the function of
transportation and avoid
excess tonification.

Applications: Irregular menstruation, functional uterine bleeding, anemia and neurasthenia.

Modifications: 1. Soreness and weakness in the lumbar region and knees. *Add:* Mulberry mistletoe (Sangjisheng), Lycium fruit (Gouqizi) and Fleece flower root (Heshouwu). 2. Indigestion and epigastric and abdominal distention and fullness. *Add:* Medicated leaven (Shenqu), Germinated barley (Maiya) and Hawthorn fruit (Shanzha). 3. Prolonged bleeding. *Add:* Donkey-hide gelatin (Ejiao), Chinese mugwort leaf (Aiye) and Antler gelatin (Lujiaojiao). 4. Edema. *Add:* Coix seed (Yiyiren) and Alisma (Zexie).

BAZHEN TANG

—Decoction of Eight Treasure Ingredients

Chinese angelica (Danggui)	10 g
Ligusticum (Chuanxiong)	5 g
White peony (Baishao)	8 g
Prepared rehmannia (Shudihuang)	15 g

Licorice (Gancao)	5 g
Ginseng (Renshen)	3 g
White atractylodes (Baizhu)	10 g
Poria (Fuling)	8 g

Method Used: Three slices of Fresh ginger (Shengjiang) and two pieces of Jujube (Dazao) added to the eight treasure ingredients are cooked with water by decoction.

Functions: To tonify *Qi* and blood.

Indications: Syndrome of *Qi* and blood deficiency.

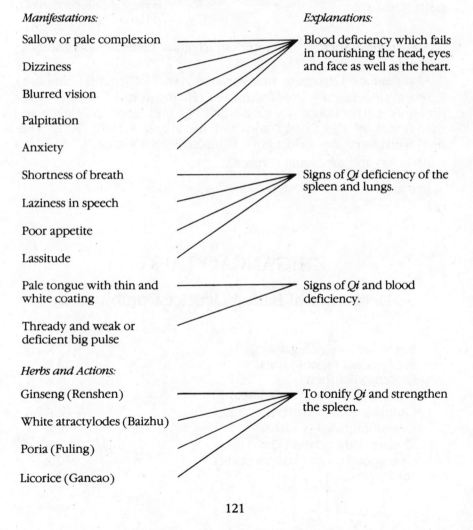

Manifestations: *Explanations:*

Sallow or pale complexion   Blood deficiency which fails in nourishing the head, eyes and face as well as the heart.

Dizziness

Blurred vision

Palpitation

Anxiety

Shortness of breath   Signs of *Qi* deficiency of the spleen and lungs.

Laziness in speech

Poor appetite

Lassitude

Pale tongue with thin and   Signs of *Qi* and blood white coating   deficiency.

Thready and weak or deficient big pulse

Herbs and Actions:

Ginseng (Renshen)   To tonify *Qi* and strengthen the spleen.

White atractylodes (Baizhu)

Poria (Fuling)

Licorice (Gancao)

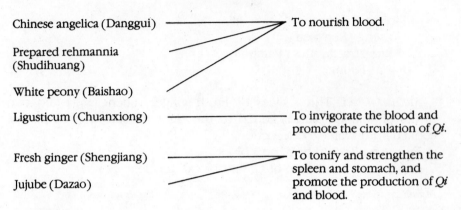

Chinese angelica (Danggui) ——————→ To nourish blood.

Prepared rehmannia
(Shudihuang)

White peony (Baishao)

Ligusticum (Chuanxiong) ————————— To invigorate the blood and
promote the circulation of *Qi*.

Fresh ginger (Shengjiang) ——————→ To tonify and strengthen the
spleen and stomach, and
Jujube (Dazao) promote the production of *Qi*
and blood.

Applications: Anemia, malnutrition, irregular menstruation and neurasthenia.

Modifications: 1. Irregular menstruation. *Add:* Motherwort (Yimucao). 2. Severe *Qi* deficiency. *Add:* Astragalus (Huangqi) and Cinnamon bark (Rougui). 3. Threatened abortion due to *Qi* and blood deficiency and dysfunction of the Chong and Ren meridians. *Replace:* Poria (Fuling) with Astragalus (Huangqi), Dipsacus root (Xuduan), Scutellaria (Huangqin) and Amomum (Sharen).

ZHIGANCAO TANG

—Decoction of Baked Licorice Combination

Baked Licorice (Zhigancao)	12 g
Fresh ginger (Shengjiang)	9 g
Ginseng (Renshen)	6 g
Fresh rehmannia (Shengdihuang)	30 g
Cannabis seed (Maziren)	10 g
Cinnamon twigs (Guizhi)	9 g
Donkey-hide gelatin (Ejiao)	9 g
Ophiopogon root (Maimendong)	10 g
Jujube (Dazao)	5-10 pcs

Method Used: Except for the Donkey-hide gelatin (Ejiao), all the other herbs are cooked with water by decoction. Then the Donkey-hide gelatin (Ejiao) is added to a cup of boiling water. Finally, these two decoctions are mixed with 10 ml of white wine.

Functions: To tonify *Qi* and replenish *Yin*.

Indications: Palpitation and intermittent pulse due to *Qi* and blood deficiency.

Manifestations:	*Explanations:*
Palpitation	Heart failing to house the mind due to blood deficiency.
Anxiety	
Irritability	
Insomnia	
Shortness of breath	Manifestations of *Qi* deficiency.
Lassitude	
Constipation	Blood deficiency and dryness in the intestines.
Pale tongue with little coating	Signs of *Qi* and blood deficiency.
Intermittent pulse or deficient, rapid pulse	

Herbs and Actions:

Baked Licorice (Zhigancao)	To tonify *Qi* and to activate circulation of *Qi* and blood.
Ginseng (Renshen)	
Donkey-hide gelatin (Ejiao)	To nourish blood and replenish *Yin*.
Dried rehmannia (Gandihuang)	
Cannabis seed (Maziren)	
Ophiopogon root (Maimendong)	

123

Cinnamon twigs (Guizhi) ——————— To invigorate heart *Yang* and promote the circulation of blood.

Jujube (Dazao) ——————— To strengthen the spleen and stomach and promote the

Fresh ginger (Shengjiang) ——————— production of *Qi* and blood.

White wine (Baijiu) ——————— To warm blood and promote its circulation, and to aid the actions of the other herbs.

Applications: Arrhythmia.

Modifications: Severe *Qi* deficiency. *Add:* Astragalus (Huangqi).

Cautions: Prolonged use of this formula may cause edema. In cases where edema exists, the dosage of Baked licorice (Zhigancao) should be reduced.

LIUWEI DIHUANG WAN

—Pills of Six Ingredients with Rehmannia Combination

Prepared rehmannia (Shudihuang)	24 g
Cornus (Shanzhuyu)	12 g
Dioscorea (Shanyao)	12 g
Poria (Fuling)	9 g
Moutan bark (Mudanpi)	9 g
Alisma (Zexie)	9 g

Method Used: The herbs are ground into powder and mixed with honey to make pills.

Functions: To replenish *Yin* in the liver and kidneys.

Indications: Yin deficiency of the liver and kidneys.

Manifestations:

Explanations:

Soreness and weakness in the lumbar region and knees ——————— *Yin* deficiency in the liver and kidneys which cannot nourish the tendons and

Heel pain ——————— bones.

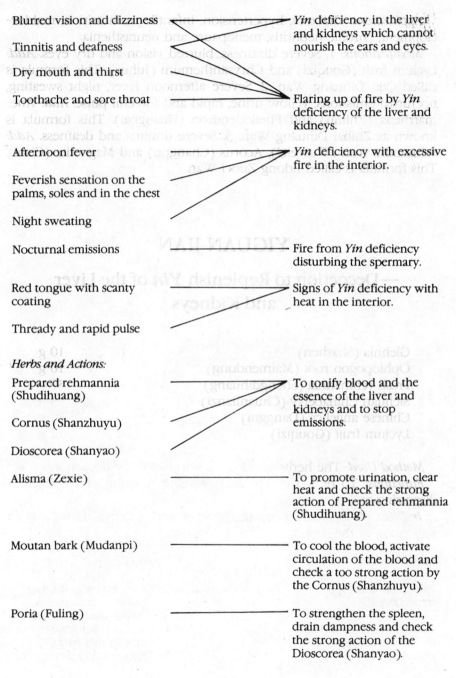

Blurred vision and dizziness

Tinnitis and deafness

Dry mouth and thirst

Toothache and sore throat

Afternoon fever

Feverish sensation on the palms, soles and in the chest

Night sweating

Nocturnal emissions

Red tongue with scanty coating

Thready and rapid pulse

Herbs and Actions:

Prepared rehmannia (Shudihuang)

Cornus (Shanzhuyu)

Dioscorea (Shanyao)

Alisma (Zexie)

Moutan bark (Mudanpi)

Poria (Fuling)

Yin deficiency in the liver and kidneys which cannot nourish the ears and eyes.

Flaring up of fire by *Yin* deficiency of the liver and kidneys.

Yin deficiency with excessive fire in the interior.

Fire from *Yin* deficiency disturbing the spermary.

Signs of *Yin* deficiency with heat in the interior.

To tonify blood and the essence of the liver and kidneys and to stop emissions.

To promote urination, clear heat and check the strong action of Prepared rehmannia (Shudihuang).

To cool the blood, activate circulation of the blood and check a too strong action by the Cornus (Shanzhuyu).

To strengthen the spleen, drain dampness and check the strong action of the Dioscorea (Shanyao).

Applications: Diabetes, hypertension, infantile malnutrition, maldevelopment, chronic nephritis, menopause and neurasthenia.

Modifications: 1. Severe dizziness, blurred vision and dry eyes. *Add:* Lycium fruit (Gouqizi) and Chrysanthemum (Juhua). This formula is called Qiju Dihuang Wan. 2. Severe afternoon fever, night sweating, nocturnal emissions, yellow urine, rapid and forceful pulse. *Add:* Anemarrhena (Zhimu) and Phellodendron (Huangbai). This formula is known as Zhibai Dihuang Wan. 3. Severe tinnitus and deafness. *Add:* Schisandra fruit (Wuweizi), Acorus (Changpu) and Magnetite (Cishi). This formula is called Erlong Zuoci Wan.

YIGUAN JIAN

—Decoction to Replenish *Yin* of the Liver and Kidneys

Glehnia (Shashen)	10 g
Ophiopogon root (Maimendong)	10 g
Fresh rehmannia (Shengdihuang)	30 g
Sichuan Chinaberry (Chuanlianzi)	5 g
Chinese angelica (Danggui)	10 g
Lycium fruit (Gouqizi)	12 g

Method Used: The herbs are cooked with water by decoction.

Functions: To replenish *Yin* and promote function of the liver in dispersing and descending.

Indications: Yin deficiency of the liver and kidneys, as well as *Qi* stagnation of the liver.

Manifestations:

Explanations:

Pain in the chest and hypochondria

Bearing down sensation of the lower abdomen and testes

Qi stagnation in the liver channels which passes through the abdomen, curving around the testes and going further to the hypochondriac region.

Epigastric pain

Bitter taste in the mouth

Acid regurgitation

Qi stagnation in the liver which transforms into fire and attacks the stomach, leading to upward perversion of the stomach *Qi*.

Dry mouth

Dry throat

Red tongue with little and dry coating

Thready and wiry or thready and weak pulse

Signs of deficiency of *Yin* blood, stagnation of *Qi* in the liver and internal heat.

Herbs and Actions:

Chinese angelica (Danggui)

To activate the blood, remove stagnation and stop pain.

Lycium fruit (Gouqizi)

Fresh rehmannia (Shengdihuang)

Ophiopogon root (Maimendong)

Glehnia (Shashen)

To nourish blood and replenish *Yin* so as to ease the liver, remove stagnation and stop pain.

Sichuan Chinaberry (Chuanlianzi)

To promote *Qi* circulation and aid the liver in dispersing and descending as well as to clear heat and stop pain.

Applications: Chronic hepatitis, chronic gastritis, gastric and duodenal ulcer, intercostal neuralgia and hernia.

Modifications: 1. Severe bitter taste in the mouth and acid regurgitation. *Add:* Coptis (Huanglian) and Evodia fruit (Wuzhuyu). 2. Constipation. *Add:* Trichosanthes (Gualou). 3. Sweating. *Add:* Wolfberry bark (Digupi). 4. Severe abdominal pain. *Add:* White peony (Baishao) and Licorice (Gancao).

127

SHENQI WAN

—Pills for Tonifying *Qi* of the Kidneys

Prepared rehmannia (Shudihuang)	240 g
Dioscorea (Shanyao)	120 g
Dogwood fruit (Shanyurou)	120 g
Alisma (Zexie)	90 g
Poria (Fuling)	90 g
Moutan bark (Mudanpi)	90 g
Cinnamon twigs (Guizhi)	30 g
Aconite (Fuzi)	30 g

Method Used: The herbs are ground into powder, then mixed with honey to make pills.

Functions: To warm and reinforce kidney *Yang*.

Indications: Kidney *Yang* deficiency.

Manifestations:

Lower back pain

Weakness of the legs

Cold feeling in the lower part of the body

Lower abdominal spasms

Impotence

Premature ejaculation

Cough and asthma due to excessive phlegm-fluid

Palpitation

Shortness of breath

Edema

Dysuria

Explanations:

Kidney *Yang* deficiency and declined fire in the Mingmen (gate of life) which cannot warm the lower *jiao*.

Yang deficiency of the kidneys which fails to control body fluids, leading to excessive phlegm-fluid to disturb the lungs and heart.

Kidney *Yang* deficiency and *Qi* dysfunction of the urinary bladder.

128

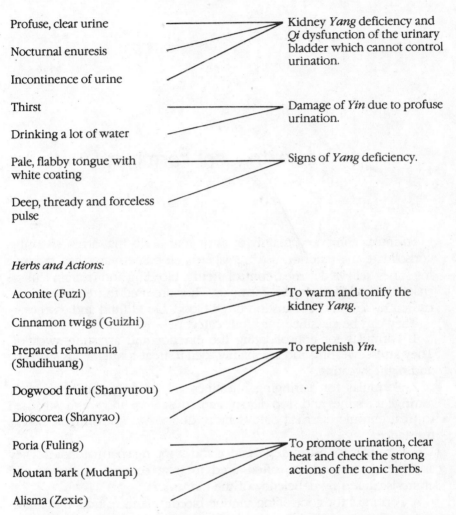

Profuse, clear urine

Nocturnal enuresis

Incontinence of urine
→ Kidney *Yang* deficiency and *Qi* dysfunction of the urinary bladder which cannot control urination.

Thirst

Drinking a lot of water
→ Damage of *Yin* due to profuse urination.

Pale, flabby tongue with white coating

Deep, thready and forceless pulse
→ Signs of *Yang* deficiency.

Herbs and Actions:

Aconite (Fuzi)

Cinnamon twigs (Guizhi)
→ To warm and tonify the kidney *Yang*.

Prepared rehmannia (Shudihuang)

Dogwood fruit (Shanyurou)

Dioscorea (Shanyao)
→ To replenish *Yin*.

Poria (Fuling)

Moutan bark (Mudanpi)

Alisma (Zexie)
→ To promote urination, clear heat and check the strong actions of the tonic herbs.

Applications: Diabetes, chronic nephritis, neurasthenia, impotence, edema and chronic bronchitis.

Modifications: Edema and dysuria. *Add:* Plantain seed (Cheqianzi) and Achyranthes (Niuxi). This formula is called Jisheng Shenqi Wan.

VII. Astringent Formulas

Formulas composed mainly of astringent herbs that arrest sweating, consolidate the exterior, astringe sperm, stop spermatorrhea, astringe intestines, relieve diarrhea, control uterine bleeding and restrain leukorrhagia are called astringent formulas. They are used to treat syndromes caused by loss and exhaustion of *Qi* blood, blood fluid and essence.

They can be classified into four categories:

1. Formulas for consolidating the exterior and arresting sweating. They arrest sweating and are mainly used to treat spontaneous sweating and night sweating.

2. Formulas for astringing intestines and stopping diarrhea. They astringe intestines and stop diarrhea and dysentery and are mostly used to treat chronic diarrhea or dysentery due to weakness in the body's resistance.

3. Formulas for astringing essence and stopping spermatorrhea. They astringe sperm and are often used to treat seminal emissions and enuresis caused by deficiency of the kidneys.

4. Formulas for controlling uterine bleeding and restraining leukorrhagia. They stop bleeding and leukorrhagia and are used for treating functional uterine bleeding as well as leukorrhagia.

Cautions: Astringent formulas are not suitable for a person with excess pathogenic factors. If they are used, the pathogenic factors will remain in the body to cause further trouble.

MULI SAN

—Powder of Oyster Shell Combination

Oyster shell (Shengmuli)	30 g
Ephedra root (Mahuanggen)	30 g
Astragalus (Huangqi)	30 g

Method Used: The herbs are cooked with water by decoction and then 30 grams of Light wheat (Fuxiaomai) are added. Or, the herbs are ground into powder.

Functions: To consolidate the exterior and astringe sweating.

Indications: Spontaneous sweating or night sweating due to *Qi* deficiency which fails in controlling the function of pores, and *Yin* deficiency which cannot astringe *Yang*.

Manifestations: *Explanations:*

Spontaneous sweating ———————— *Qi* deficiency which fails in controlling the function of pores.

Night sweating ———————— *Yin* deficiency which makes *Yang Qi* flow out.

Shortness of breath ———————— *Qi* deficiency.

Palpitation

Irritability

The heart and mind disturbed by *Yin* deficiency with heat in the interior.

Light red tongue

Thready and weak pulse

Signs of deficiency of *Qi* and blood.

Herbs and Actions:

Oyster shell (Shengmuli)

Light wheat (Fuxiaomai)

To astringe *Yin*, subside *Yang*, clear heat and relieve irritability.

Ephedra root (Mahuanggen) ———————— To stop sweating.

Astragalus (Huangqi) ———————— To promote *Qi*.

Applications: Spontaneous sweating, night sweating and prolonged, profuse perspiration due to weakness of the body.

Modifications: 1. *Yang* deficiency manifested by severe spontaneous sweating. *Add:* White atractylodes (Baizhu) and Aconite (Fuzi). 2. *Yin* deficiency manifested by severe night sweating. *Add:* White peony (Baishao), Dried rehmannia (Gandihuang) and Wild jujube seed (Suanzaoren). 3. Severe blood deficiency. *Add:* Prepared rehmannia (Shudihuang) and Donkey-hide gelatin (Ejiao). 4. Severe *Qi* deficiency. *Add:* Pilose asiabell root (Dangshen) and White atractylodes (Baizhu).

Cautions: For a person with night sweating caused by *Yin* deficiency and excessive fire in the interior or for a person with profuse sweating, cold limbs and weak pulse due to collapse of *Yang*, the formula should not be used alone.

YUPINGFENG SAN

—The Jade Screen Powder

Ledebouriella root (Fangfeng)	30 g
White atractylodes (Baizhu)	60 g
Astragalus (Huangqi)	30 g

Method Used: The herbs are ground into powder.

Functions: 1. To tonify *Qi* and consolidate the exterior. 2. To stop sweating.

Indications: Spontaneous sweating due to exterior deficiency.

Manifestations:

Explanations:

Spontaneous sweating

Aversion to wind

Deficiency of the defensive *Qi* which cannot protect the exterior, but makes pores open.

Pale complexion

Pale tongue with thin and white coating

Deficient and forceless pulse

Signs of *Qi* deficiency.

Herbs and Actions:

Astragalus (Huangqi) ————————→ To tonify *Qi*, consolidate the
                                       exterior and stop sweating.

White atractylodes (Baizhu)

Ledebouriella root (Fangfeng)————————— To dispel wind and release
                                        the exterior.

Applications: Spontaneous sweating due to weakness of the body.

Modifications: 1. Severe spontaneous sweating. *Add:* Light wheat (Fuxiaomai), Oyster shell (Shengmuli) and Schisandra fruit (Wuweizi). 2. Allergic rhinitis. *Add:* Magnolia flower (Xinyihua), Angelica (Baizhi) and Xanthium fruit (Cangerzi).

Cautions: For a patient with wind-cold-exterior-deficiency syndrome manifested by fever, sweating, aversion to wind and tardy pulse, the formula should not be used; rather Guizhi Tang is suggested.

JINSUO GUJING WAN

—Pills to Fix Sperm

Flattened milkvetch seed (Shayuanjili)	60 g
Euryale seed (Qianshi)	60 g
Dragon's bone (Longgu)	30 g
Lotus seed (Lianzirou)	60 g
Lotus stamen (Lianzixu)	60 g
Oyster shell (Shengmuli)	30 g

Method Used: The herbs and substances are made into pills which can be taken with salted boiling water.

Functions: To reinforce the kidneys and astringe the essence.

Indications: Nocturnal and spontaneous emissions caused by kidney deficiency which cannot control (sperm) essence.

Manifestations: *Explanations:*

Nocturnal and spontaneous ————————— Kidney deficiency which fails
emissions   in controlling the essence.

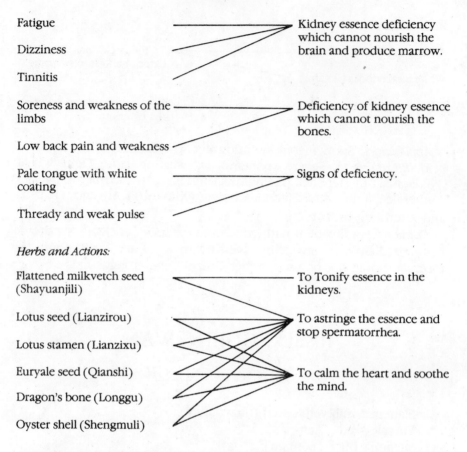

Fatigue — Kidney essence deficiency which cannot nourish the brain and produce marrow.

Dizziness

Tinnitis

Soreness and weakness of the limbs — Deficiency of kidney essence which cannot nourish the bones.

Low back pain and weakness

Pale tongue with white coating — Signs of deficiency.

Thready and weak pulse

Herbs and Actions:

Flattened milkvetch seed (Shayuanjili) — To Tonify essence in the kidneys.

Lotus seed (Lianzirou) — To astringe the essence and stop spermatorrhea.

Lotus stamen (Lianzixu)

Euryale seed (Qianshi) — To calm the heart and soothe the mind.

Dragon's bone (Longgu)

Oyster shell (Shengmuli)

Applications: Neurasthenia.

Modifications: 1. *Yin* deficiency with excessive fire and flaring up of Mingmen (gate of life) fire. *Add:* Anemarrhena (Zhimu) and Phellodendron (Huangbai). 2. Kidney *Yin* deficiency with internal heat. *Add:* Tortoise plastron (Guiban) and Ligustrum fruit (Nüzhenzi). 3. Deficiency of the kidney *Yang*. *Add:* Dogwood fruit (Shanyurou) and Psoralea (Buguzhi). 4. Constipation. *Add:* Cistanche (Roucongrong) and Chinese angelica (Danggui). 5. Loose stool. *Add:* Schisandra fruit (Wuweizi) and Psoralea (Buguzhi). 6. Severe low back pain and soreness. *Add:* Eucommia bark (Duzhong), Dipsacus root (Xuduan) and Mulberry mistletoe (Sangjisheng). 7. Impotence and premature ejaculation. *Add:* Epimedium (Yinyanghuo), Cynomorium (Suoyang) and Dodder seed (Tusizi).

134

SISHEN WAN

—Pills of Four Miraculous Ingredients

Nutmeg (Roudoukou)	60 g
Schisandra fruit (Wuweizi)	60 g
Psoralea (Buguzhi)	120 g
Evodia fruit (Wuzhuyu)	30 g

Method Used: The ingredients are ground into powder along with 240 grams of Fresh ginger (Shengjiang) and 100 pieces of Jujube (Dazao), then made into pills.

Functions: 1. To warm and reinforce the spleen and kidneys. 2. To astringe intestines and stop diarrhea.

Indications: Morning diarrhea or chronic diarrhea caused by weakness and coldness in the spleen and kidneys.

Manifestations:

Explanations:

Morning diarrhea ———————— Deficiency of the kidney *Yang* and the declined fire of Mingmen (gate of life).

Chronic diarrhea ———————— *Yang* deficiency of the spleen and kidneys.

Abdominal pain ———————— Coldness in the spleen and kidneys, leading to *Qi* stagnation.

Loss of appetite ————————

Indigestion ———————— *Yang* deficiency of the spleen and stomach which cannot digest and absorb food and drink.

Soreness of the lower back ————————

Cold limbs ———————— Deficiency of the spleen and kidneys which cannot nourish the bones and muscles.

Weakness of the limbs ————————

Fatigue ———————— *Yang Qi* deficiency.

Pale tongue with white and thin coating ─────────────→ Signs of deficiency and coldness.

Deep, slow and forceless pulse

Herbs and Actions:

Psoralea (Buguzhi) ───────────── To warm and reinforce kidney *Yang.*

Evodia fruit (Wuzhuyu) ───────── To warm the middle *jiao* and dispel coldness.

Nutmeg (Roudoukou)

Schisandra fruit (Wuweizi) ────── To astringe intestines and stop diarrhea.

Fresh ginger (Shengjiang) ─────── To strengthen the spleen and stomach.

Jujube (Dazao)

Applications: Chronic enteritis and intestinal tuberculosis.

Modifications: 1. Prolapse of rectum. *Add:* Astragalus (Huangqi), Cimicifuga (Shengma) and Pilose asiabell root (Dangshen). 2. Severe soreness of the lower back and cold limbs. *Add:* Aconite (Fuzi) and Cinnamon bark (Rougui).

GUCHONG TANG

—Decoction to Consolidate the Chong Channel

White atractylodes (Baizhu)	30 g
White peony (Baishao)	12 g
Dragon's bone (Longgu)	24 g
Dogwood fruit (Shanyurou)	24 g
Cuttlefish bone (Wuzeigu)	12 g
Carbonized petiole (Zonglütan)	9 g
Schisandra fruit (Wuweizi)	1.5 g
Astragalus (Huangqi)	18 g
Oyster shell (Shengmuli)	24 g
Rubia root (Qiancao)	9 g

Method Used: The herbs and substance are cooked with water by decoction.

Functions: 1. To tonify *Qi* and strengthen the spleen. 2. To consolidate the Chong channel and control the blood.

Indications: Menorrhagia or uterine bleeding due to weakness of the spleen and stomach, deficiency of *Qi* and blood and the unconsolidated Chong channel.

Manifestations:	*Explanations:*
Menorrhagia or uterine bleeding	Deficiency of *Qi* and blood and the unconsolidated Chong channel which cannot control the blood.
Light red and dilute menstruation flow	Signs of deficiency of *Qi* and blood.
Palpitation	
Shortness of breath	
Pale tongue with thin and white coating	
Thready and weak or deficient and big pulse	

Herbs and Actions:

Astragalus (Huangqi)	To tonify *Qi*, strengthen the spleen, control the blood, consolidate the Chong channel and stop bleeding.
White atractylodes (Baizhu)	
White peony (Baishao)	To replenish *Yin* and nourish blood.
Dogwood fruit (Shanyurou)	
Dragon's bone (Longgu)	To astringe and stop bleeding.
Oyster shell (Shengmuli)	
Cuttlefish bone (Wuzeigu)	
Schisandra fruit (Wuweizi)	
Carbonized petiole (Zonglütan)	

Rubia root (Qiancao) ———————— To invigorate blood circulation and remove stagnation.

Applications: Menorrhagia, functional uterine bleeding and postpartum hemorrhage.

Modifications: Listlessness, pale complexion, cold limbs and weak pulse. *Add:* Ginseng (Renshen) and Aconite (Fuzi).

WANDAI TANG

—Decoction to Treat Leukorrhagia

White atractylodes (Baizhu)	30 g
Dioscorea (Shanyao)	30 g
Ginseng (Renshen)	6 g
White peony (Baishao)	15 g
Plantain seed (Cheqianzi)	9 g
Schizonepeta (Jingjie)	1.5 g
Atractylodes rhizome (Cangzhu)	9 g
Licorice (Gancao)	3 g
Citrus peel (Jupi)	1.5 g
Bupleurum (Chaihu)	1.8 g

Method Used: The herbs are cooked with water by decoction.

Functions: 1. To reinforce the middle *jiao* and strengthen the spleen. 2. To resolve dampness and relieve leukorrhagia.

Indications: Leukorrhagia due to flowing downward of the turbid dampness by deficiency of the spleen and *Qi* stagnation of the liver.

Manifestations:	*Explanations:*
White, clear and dilute leukorrhagia with no offensive smell	Unconsolidated Chong channel and flowing downward of turbid dampness by deficiency of the spleen and *Qi* stagnation of the liver.

Loose stool ———————————— Excessive dampness from deficiency of the spleen.

Fatigue ———————————— Qi deficiency and weakness of the spleen.

Pale complexion

Pale tongue with white coating ———————————— Signs of Qi deficiency, excessive dampness and weakness of the spleen.

Tardy or soft and weak pulse

Herbs and Actions:

Ginseng (Renshen) ———————————— To tonify Qi and strengthen the spleen.

White atractylodes (Baizhu)

Dioscorea (Shanyao)

Atractylodes rhizome (Cangzhu) ———————————— To regulate Qi, strengthen the spleen and dry dampness.

Citrus peel (Jupi)

Plantain seed (Cheqianzi) ———————————— To promote urination and drain dampness.

White peony (Baishao) ———————————— To ease the liver and remove stagnation.

Bupleurum (Chaihu) ———————————— To uplift Yang Qi and stop the downward flow of the turbid dampness.

Schizonepeta (Jingjie) ———————————— To dispel wind and eliminate dampness.

Licorice (Gancao) ———————————— To harmonize actions of the other herbs.

Applications: Leukorrhagia, vulvitis, vaginitis and cervical inflammation.

Modifications: 1. Soreness and pain in the lower back. *Add:* Eucommia bark (Duzhong), Dodder seed (Tusizi) and Dipsacus root (Xuduan). 2. Abdominal pain. *Add:* Chinese mugwort leaf (Aiye), Cyperus tuber (Xiangfu) and Lindera root (Wuyao). 3. Prolonged deficiency and coldness. *Add:* Deglued antler powder (Lujiaoshuang), Cinnamon bark (Rougui), Morinda root (Bajitian) and Cuttlefish bone (Wuzeigu).

YIHUANG TANG

—Decoction to Treat Yellow Leukorrhagia

Dioscorea (Shanyao)	30 g
Euryale seed (Qianshi)	30 g
Plantain seed (Cheqianzi)	3 g
Ginkgo seed (Baiguo)	10 pcs
Phellodendron (Huangbai)	6 g

Method Used: The herbs are cooked with water by decoction.

Functions: 1. To strengthen the spleen and dry dampness. 2. To clear heat and relieve leukorrhagia.

Indications: Leukorrhagia due to damp-heat in the interior.

Manifestations:

Explanations:

Yellow, sticky leukorrhagia with offensive smell —————— Deficiency of the spleen, producing dampness which transforms into heat; the downward flow of damp-heat, causing yellow leukorrhagia.

Heavy sensation in the head ——————

Dizziness and vertigo —————— Deficiency of the spleen which brings about excessive dampness, impairing the ascending of the clean *Yang*.

Fatigue —————— *Qi* deficiency and weakness of the spleen.

Pale tongue with white coating ——————

Soft or rapid pulse —————— Signs of spleen deficiency and excessive damp-heat in the interior.

140

Herbs and Actions:

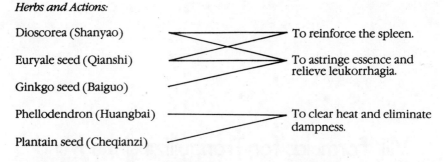

Dioscorea (Shanyao)

Euryale seed (Qianshi)

Ginkgo seed (Baiguo)

Phellodendron (Huangbai)

Plantain seed (Cheqianzi)

To reinforce the spleen.

To astringe essence and relieve leukorrhagia.

To clear heat and eliminate dampness.

Applications: Yellow leukorrhagia, vulvitis, vaginitis and cervical inflammation.

Modifications: 1. Severe damp-heat. *Add:* Chinese gentiana (Longdancao) and Capejasmine fruit (Zhizi). 2. Depressed liver manifested by irritability and hot temper. *Add:* Bupleurum (Chaihu) and White peony (Baishao).

VIII. Formulas for Tranquilizing the Mind

Formulas used as sedatives and tranquilizers that treat emotional distress and morbid fear and distrust are called tranquilizing formulas. They can be classified into two categories:

1. Formulas for nourishing the heart and calming the mind. They nourish blood and soothe the mind, and are used to treat disturbances of the mind syndromes caused by deficiency of blood in the heart.

2. Formulas for calming the heart and tranquilizing the mind. They tranquilize the mind, and are used to treat excess type syndromes of disturbances of the mind. This group of formulas composed of toxic mineral drugs cannot be taken for long periods of time.

ZHUSHA ANSHEN WAN

—Pills to Soothe the Mind with Cinnabar Combination

Cinnabar (Zhusha)	15 g
Coptis (Huanglian)	18 g
Licorice (Gancao)	16 g
Fresh rehmannia (Shengdihuang)	8 g
Chinese angelica (Danggui)	8 g

Method Used: The herbs and substances are ground into powder, then made into pills.

Functions: 1. To calm the heart and soothe the mind. 2. To reduce fire and replenish *Yin.*

Indications: Disturbance of the mind by the flaring up of fire due to deficiency of *Yin* and blood.

Manifestations:	*Explanations:*
Insomnia	Mind disturbed by flaring up of the heart fire which consumes *Yin* and blood.
Dreamful sleep	
Palpitations	
Anxiety	
Irritability	
Nausea	Perversion of the stomach *Qi* which goes up together with the fire.
Red tongue with little coating	Signs of *Yin* deficiency with heat in the interior.
Thready and rapid pulse	

Herbs and Actions:

Cinnabar (Zhusha)	To calm the heart and soothe the mind.
Coptis (Huanglian)	To clear heat in the heart and relieve irritability.
Fresh rehmannia (Shengdihuang)	
Chinese angelica (Danggui)	To replenish *Yin* and nourish blood.
Licorice (Gancao)	To harmonize actions of the other herbs.

Applications: Neurasthenia.

Cautions: As Cinnabar (Zhusha) in the formula is toxic, over dosages or prolonged use of the pills is not suggested.

SUANZAOREN TANG

—Decoction of Wild Jujube Seed Combination

Wild jujube seed (Suanzaoren)	15-18 g
Licorice (Gancao)	3 g
Anemarrhena (Zhimu)	8-10 g
Ligusticum (Chuanxiong)	3-5 g
Poria (Fuling)	10 g

Method Used: Wild jujube seed (Suanzaoren) are well boiled, then added to the other herbs and cooked by decoction.

Functions: 1. To nourish the blood and soothe the mind. 2. To clear heat and relieve irritability.

Indications: Disturbance of the mind by hyperfunction of the liver due to deficiency of blood.

Manifestations:

Palpitations

Anxiety

Irritability

Insomnia

Night sweating

Dizziness

Vertigo or distention and pain in the head

Blurred vision

Dry mouth and throat

Thready, wiry and rapid pulse

Explanations:

Disturbance of the mind caused by flaring up of the heart fire derived from blood deficiency.

Blood deficiency and heat in the interior.

Head and eyes attacked by hyperfunction of *Yang* of the liver due to blood deficiency.

Signs of *Yin* deficiency with heat in the interior.

144

Herbs and Actions:

Wild jujube seed
(Suanzaoren) ——————————— To astringe sweating and
promote the production of
body fluids.

Poria (Fuling) ——————————— To calm the heart and soothe
the mind.

Anemarrhena (Zhimu) ——————————— To replenish *Yin*, clear heat
and relieve irritability.

Ligusticum (Chuanxiong) ——————————— To invigorate blood
circulation, promote *Qi*, ease
the liver and remove
stagnation.

Licorice (Gancao) ——————————— To harmonize actions of the
other herbs.

Applications: Neurasthenia, paroxysmal tachycardia and climacteric syndrome.

Modifications: 1. Severe *Yin* deficiency and internal heat. *Add:* White peony (Baishao) and Fresh rehmannia (Shengdihuang). 2. Severe night sweating. *Add:* Schisandra fruit (Wuweizi). 3. Severe palpitation and anxiety. *Add:* Dragon's bone (Longgu) and Oyster shell (Shengmuli).

TIANWANG BUXIN DAN

—The Heavenly King's Tonic Pills

Fresh rehmannia (Shengdihuang)	12 g
Ginseng (Renshen)	15 g
Scrophularia (Xuanshen)	15 g
Schisandra fruit (Wuweizi)	15 g
Platycodon (Jiegeng)	15 g
Asparagus root (Tianmendong)	60 g
Ophiopogon root (Maimendong)	60 g
Wild jujube seed (Suanzaoren)	60 g
Red sage root (Danshen)	15 g

Poria (Fuling)	15 g
Polygala root (Yuanzhi)	15 g
Chinese angelica (Danggui)	60 g
Biota seed (Baiziren)	60 g

Method Used: The powders of the herbs are mixed with honey and made into pills coated with 5-15 grams of Cinnabar (Zhusha).

Functions: 1. To replenish *Yin* and nourish blood. 2. To tonify the heart and soothe the mind.

Indications: Disturbance of the mind by *Yin* and blood deficiency of the heart and kidneys.

Manifestations:

Explanations:

Palpitations

Anxiety

Irritability

Insomnia

Fatigue

Forgetfulness

Disturbance of the mind by attack of fire due to *Yin* and blood deficiency in the heart and kidneys.

Night sweating ———— *Yin* deficiency with heat in the interior.

Nocturnal emissions ———— The chamber of sperm attacked by extravasation of the Minister Fire (in kidneys) and the mind disturbed by the flaring up of fire in the interior.

Constipation ———— Blood deficiency and dryness in the intestines.

Ulceration of the mouth and tongue ———— Flaring up of fire due to *Yin* and blood deficiency.

Red tongue with little coating

Thready and rapid pulse

Signs of *Yin* deficiency with heat in the interior.

146

Herbs and Actions:

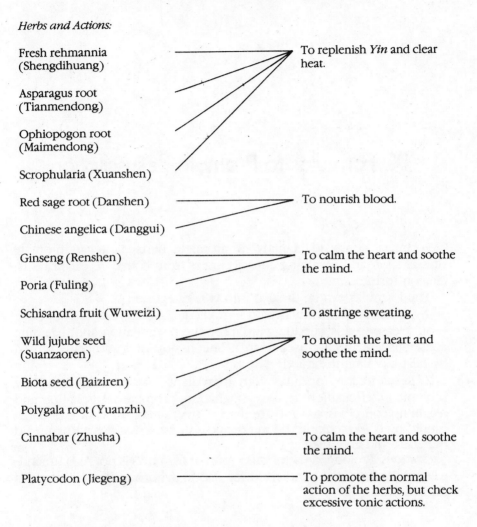

Fresh rehmannia
(Shengdihuang)

Asparagus root
(Tianmendong)

Ophiopogon root
(Maimendong)

Scrophularia (Xuanshen)

To replenish *Yin* and clear heat.

Red sage root (Danshen)

Chinese angelica (Danggui)

To nourish blood.

Ginseng (Renshen)

Poria (Fuling)

To calm the heart and soothe the mind.

Schisandra fruit (Wuweizi)

To astringe sweating.

Wild jujube seed
(Suanzaoren)

Biota seed (Baiziren)

Polygala root (Yuanzhi)

To nourish the heart and soothe the mind.

Cinnabar (Zhusha)

To calm the heart and soothe the mind.

Platycodon (Jiegeng)

To promote the normal action of the herbs, but check excessive tonic actions.

Applications: Neurasthenia and paroxysmal tachycardia.

IX. Formulas to Promote Resuscitation

Formulas composed chiefly of aromatic herbs that can promote resuscitation and regaining consciousness from coma are called resuscitation formulas.

The formulas can be divided into two categories.

1. Resuscitation formulas with ingredients of cold nature. They clear heat, release toxins, subdue wind, promote resuscitation and regaining consciousness and are used to treat unconsciousness and coma caused by heat blocking the mind.

2. Resuscitation formulas with ingredients of warm nature. They promote *Qi* circulation, remove stagnation, promote resuscitation and regaining consciousness and are used to treat unconsciousness or coma caused by cold blocking the mind, and stifling sensations and pains in the chest and abdomen.

Cautions: Prolonged use of this group of formulas is not recommended, and they are contraindicated for flaccid syndromes with coma and unconsciousness.

The following table is a comparison of functions among Ox Gallstone Resurrection Pills (Angong Niuhuang Wan), Most Precious Pellets (Zhibao Dan), Purple Snowy Powder (Zixue Dan) and Styrax Pills (Suhexiang Wan):

	Ox Gallstone Resurrection Pills (Angong Niuhuang Wan)	The Most Precious Pellets (Zhibao Dan)	Purple Snowy Powder (Zixue Dan)	Styrax Pills (Suhexiang Wan)
To clear heat and release toxins	+++	+	++	0
To promote resuscitation	++	+++	++	+++
To eliminate wind and stop convulsions	+	+	+++	0
To resolve phlegm	+	+	0	+
To promote Qi and remove stagnation	0	0	0	+++
To regulate bowel movements	0	0	+	0
Property	cool	cool	cool	warm

From the table, we see that all the formulas except the last one have the functions of clearing heat, releasing toxins, promoting resuscitation and eliminating endogenous wind, but they are different in intensity. Ox Gallstone Resurrection Pills (Angong Niuhuang Wan) are the most powerful for clearing heat and releasing toxins and are used to treat febrile diseases due to invasion by exogenous pathogenic factors. They are used to treat high fever, loss of consciousness, coma as well as convulsions; Most Precious Pellets (Zhibao Dan) are strong in promoting resuscitation, but poor in clearing heat and releasing toxins. They

149

can relieve sudden coma. Purple Snowy Powder (Zixue Dan) in the aspect of clearing heat and releasing toxins is not as good as Ox gallstone resurrection pills, (Angong Niuhuang Wan), but better than Most Precious Pellets (Zhibao Dan); in promoting resuscitation, it is not as good as Most Precious Pellets (Zhibao Dan), but is similar to Ox Gallstone Resurrection Pills (Angong Niuhuang Wan). Purple Snowy Powder (Zixue Dan) is the strongest one among the four formulas in eliminating endogenous wind and stopping convulsions, regulating bowel movements and dispelling heat. They are mostly used in febrile diseases manifested by high fever, loss of consciousness, coma, convulsions and constipation. Styrax Pills (Suhexiang Wan) have the more powerful functions of promoting resuscitation, promoting *Qi* and resolving stagnation. It is often used in extravasation of *Qi* and retention of turbid phlegm. The manifestations are sudden coma, stifling sensations and colic pain in the chest and abdomen like angina pectoralgia.

X. Qi Formulas

Formulas that regulate the flow of *Qi* and treat dysfunction of *Qi* are called *Qi* formulas. They can be divided into two categories:

1. Formulas for promoting *Qi* circulation. They promotes *Qi* circulation and remove stagnation and are used to treat syndromes caused by *Qi* stagnation in the liver or in the spleen and stomach.

2. Formulas for descending *Qi*. They conduct *Qi* downward and are used to treat syndromes caused by upward perversion of *Qi* of the lungs or stomach.

YUE JU WAN

—Pills to Remove Stagnation

Atractylodes rhizome (Cangzhu)	15 g
Cyperus tuber (Xiangfu)	15 g
Ligusticum (Chuanxiong)	15 g
Medicated leaven (Shenqu)	15 g
Capejasmine fruit (Zhizi)	15 g

Method Used: The herbs are ground into powder, and then mixed with water and made into pills.

Functions: To promote *Qi* and remove stagnation.

Indications: Stagnation of *Qi*, stagnation of blood, accumulation of fire, accumulation of dampness, retention of food and retention of phlegm.

Manifestations: *Explanations:*

Stifling sensation and fullness —————————— *Qi* stagnation, blood
in the chest and diaphragm   stagnation and a depressed
                                                     liver.
Hypochondriac pain

Distention and fullness in
epigastric and abdominal
regions

Acid regurgitation   —————————— Dysfunction of the stomach
                                                     in descending caused by
Vomiting   attack of the liver fire.

Indigestion   —————————— *Qi* stagnation, retention of
                                                     food and accumulation of
                                                     dampness and phlegm in the
                                                     stomach.

Herbs and Actions:

Cyperus tuber (Xiangfu)   —————————— To promote *Qi* in the liver
                                                     and remove stagnation.

Ligusticum (Chuanxiong)   —————————— To invigorate blood and
                                                     promote *Qi*.

Capejasmine fruit (Zhizi)   —————————— To clear heat and conduct
                                                     fire downward.

Atractylodes rhizome   —————————— To dry dampness and
(Cangzhu)   strengthen the spleen and
                                                     stomach.

Medicated leaven (Shenqu)   —————————— To harmonize the stomach
                                                     for digestion.

152

Applications: Chronic gastritis, gastric or duodenal ulcer, irregular menstruation, intercostal neuralgia, dysmenorrhea and cholecystitis.

Modifications: 1. Severe *Qi* stagnation. *Add:* Costus root (Muxiang), Bitter orange (Zhiqiao), Green tangerine peel (Qingpi) and Citrus peel (Jupi). 2. Severe blood stagnation. *Add:* Peach seed (Taoren), Carthamus (Honghua), Red sage root (Danshen) and Chinese angelica (Danggui). 3. Severe accumulation of fire. *Add:* Coptis (Huanglian), Natural indigo (Qingdai) and Forsythia (Lianqiao). 4. Severe accumulation of dampness. *Add:* Poria (Fuling), Alisma (Zexie), Plantain seed (Cheqianzi) and Coix seed (Yiyiren). 5. Retention of food. *Add:* Hawthorn fruit (Shanzha), Germinated barley (Maiya), Chicken's gizzard skin (Jineijin), and Carbonized areca seed (Jiaobinglang). 6. Excessive phlegm. *Add:* Trichosanthes (Gualou), Arisaema with bile (Dannanxing) and Pinellia tuber (Banxia). 7. Cold manifestations. *Add:* Evodia fruit (Wuzhuyu), Galanga (Gaoliangjiang) and Dried ginger (Ganjiang). 8. Dysmenorrhea. *Add:* Curcuma root (Yujin), Motherwort (Yimucao), Chinese angelica (Danggui) and White peony (Baishao).

Cautions: The formula is contraindicated in any deficiency syndromes.

LIANG FU WAN

—Pills of Galanga and Cyperus Tuber

Galanga (Gaoliangjiang)	15 g
Cyperus tuber (Xiangfu)	15 g

Method Used: The two herbs are ground into powder, mixed with Fresh ginger juice (Shengjiangzhi) and made into pills.

Functions: 1. To promote *Qi* in the liver. 2. To dispel cold and stop pain.

Indications: Pain in the epigastric, abdominal and hypochondriac regions caused by *Qi* stagnation and coldness.

Manifestations:

Epigastric pain

Stifling in chest

Hypochondriac pain

Menorrhagia

Explanations:

Qi stagnation in the liver and stomach.

Pale tongue with white coating

Deep, wiry or choppy pulse

Signs of retardation of circulation of Qi and blood as well as coldness in the interior.

Herbs and Actions:

Galanga (Gaoliangjiang)

Fresh ginger juice (Shengjiangzhi)

To warm the middle *jiao* and dispel cold.

Cyperus tuber (Xiangfu)

To promote Qi in the liver and stop pain.

Applications: Chronic gastritis, gastrospasms, gastric or duodenal ulcer, gastroneurosis, irregular menstruation, chronic hepatitis and intercostal neuralgia.

Modifications: 1. Severe Qi deficiency. Double dosage of Cyperus tuber (Xiangfu); or add Costus root (Muxiang) and Lindera root (Wuyao) or Citrus peel (Jupi) and Bitter orange (Zhiqiao). 2. Severe coldness in the interior. Double dosage of Galanga (Gaoliangjiang); or add Evodia fruit (Wuzhuyu) and Dried ginger (Ganjiang). 3. Hypochondriac pain. *Add:* Green Tangerine peel (Qingpi). 4. Epigastric pain. *Add:* Costus root (Muxiang). 5. Menorrhagia. *Add:* Chinese angelica (Danggui) and Ligusticum (Chuanxiong).

Cautions: It is contraindicated in any pain due to heat in the interior.

JINLINGZI SAN

—Powder of Sichuan Chinaberry Combination

Sichuan chinaberry (Chuanlianzi)	30 g
Corydalis tuber (Yanhusuo)	30 g

Method Used: The herbs are ground into powder which is taken with wine or boiling water.

Functions: 1. To promote *Qi* in the liver. 2. To invigorate blood and stop pain.

Indications: Pain in the chest, abdominal and hypochondriac regions caused by fire due to *Qi* stagnation in the liver.

Manifestations: *Explanations:*

Pain in the chest, abdominal ———————— Stagnation of *Qi* and blood in
and hypochondriac regions   the liver.

Dysmenorrhea

Hernia pain

Red tongue with yellow ———————— Signs of prolonged liver *Qi*
coating   stagnation transforming into
                                                   fire.
Wiry and rapid pulse

Herbs and Actions:

Corydalis tuber (Yanhusuo) ———————— To invigorate blood and
                                            promote *Qi* so as to stop pain.

Sichuan chinaberry ———————— To promote *Qi* in the liver,
(Chuanlianzi)   stop pain and reduce heat.

Applications: Chronic hepatitis, irregular menstruation, hernia and intercostal neuralgia.

Modifications: 1. Severe dysmenorrhea. *Add:* Moutan bark (Mudanpi), Motherwort (Yimucao), Red peony (Chishao) and Cyperus tuber (Xiangfu). 2. Hernia pain. *Add:* Tangerine seed (Juhe). If the hernia pain is caused by cold, add Fennel fruit (Xiaohuixiang) and Evodia fruit (Wuzhuyu).

Cautions: 1. The formula is contraindicated during pregnancy. 2. The powder should not be used for a person with pain caused by cold.

BANXIA HOUPO TANG

—Decoction of Pinellia Tuber and Magnolia Bark Combination

Pinellia tuber (Banxia)	12 g
Magnolia bark (Houpo)	9 g
Fresh ginger (Shengjiang)	9 g
Perilla leaf (Zisuye)	6 g
Poria (Fuling)	12 g

Method Used: The herbs are cooked with water by decoction.

Functions: 1. To promote *Qi* and remove nodules. 2. To conduct perversion and resolve phlegm.

Indications: Globus hystericus caused by phlegm associated with *Qi* stagnation in the liver and impairment of body fluid distribution.

Manifestations:

Explanations:

A sensation of a foreign body in the throat

Stifling sensation and fullness in the chest and hypochondriac region

Cough with profuse white sputum

Nausea

Vomiting

Phlegm associated with stagnation of *Qi* in the throat, chest, epigastric and hypochondriac regions.

156

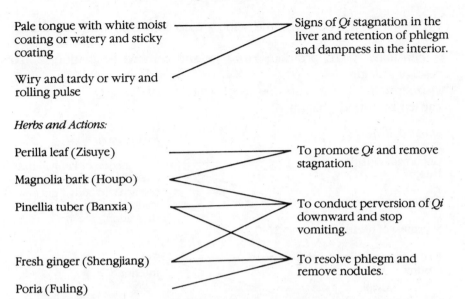

Pale tongue with white moist coating or watery and sticky coating ——————→ Signs of *Qi* stagnation in the liver and retention of phlegm and dampness in the interior.

Wiry and tardy or wiry and rolling pulse

Herbs and Actions:

Perilla leaf (Zisuye) ——————→ To promote *Qi* and remove stagnation.

Magnolia bark (Houpo)

Pinellia tuber (Banxia) ——————→ To conduct perversion of *Qi* downward and stop vomiting.

Fresh ginger (Shengjiang) ——————→ To resolve phlegm and remove nodules.

Poria (Fuling)

Applications: Neurasthenia and chronic pharyngitis.

Modifications: 1. Severe distention and fullness in the chest and hypochondriac region. *Add:* Bupleurum (Chaihu), Cyperus tuber tuber (Xiangfu), White peony (Baishao) and Curcuma root (Yujin). 2. Red tongue with white and little moist coating. *Add:* Glehnia (Shashen), Ophiopogon root (Maimendong) and Scrophularia (Xuanshen). 3. If Jujube (Dazao) is added to the formula, there is no difference in indication, but the formula with Jujube (Dazao) is milder.

GUALOU XIEBAI BAIJIU TANG

—Decoction of Trichosanthes, Macrostem Onion and White Wine Combination

Trichosanthes (Gualou)	12 g
Macrostem Onion (Xiebai)	12 g
White Wine (Baijiu)	30 cc

Method Used: The herbs and wine are cooked with water by decoction.

Functions: 1. To promote *Yang Qi* and remove stagnation. 2. To resolve phlegm.

Indications: Chest pain due to obstruction of *Yang Qi* in the chest caused by turbid phlegm.

Manifestations:

Explanations:

Chest pain radiating to the back

Stifling sensation in the chest

Shortness of breath

Dysfunction of *Yang* in the chest which cannot distribute essence and body fluids, leading to phlegm and *Qi* stagnation.

Pale tongue with white sticky coating

Deep and wiry or tight pulse

Signs of cold-phlegm in the interior.

Herbs and Actions:

Trichosanthes (Gualou)

To resolve phlegm.

To ease the chest and remove stagnation.

Macrostem onion (Xiebai)

To regulate *Yang Qi.*

White wine (Baijiu)

To promote *Qi*, invigorate blood circulation and aid the actions of the other herbs in regulating *Yang Qi* and removing stagnation.

Applications: Angina pectoris and intercostal neuralgia.

Modifications: 1. Severe angina pectoris. *Add:* Red sage root (Danshen), Red peony (Chishao), Carthamus (Honghua) and Ligusticum (Chuanxiong). 2. Attack by severe pathogenic cold. *Add:* Cinnamon twigs (Guizhi) and Dried ginger (Ganjiang). 3. Blockage by turbid phlegm. *Add:* Pinellia tuber (Banxia) and Fresh ginger (Shengjiang). 4. Severe stifling sensation in the chest. *Add:* Immature bitter orange (Zhishi) or Bitter orange (Zhiqiao) and Magnolia bark (Houpo).

TIANTAI WUYAO SAN

—Powder of Lindera Root from Tiantai

Lindera root (Wuyao)	12 g
Costus root (Muxiang)	6 g
Fennel fruit (Xiaohuixiang)	6 g
Green tangerine peel (Qingpi)	6 g
Galanga (Gaoliangjiang)	9 g
Areca seed (Binglang)	9 g
Sichuan chinaberry (Chuanlianzi)	12 g
Croton seed (Badou)	70 pcs

Method Used: Croton seed (Badou) and Sichuan chinaberry (Chuanlianzi) are carbonized. The carbonized Sichuan chinaberry (Chuanlianzi) with the above ingredients and water are cooked by decoction. Then yellow wine is added to the decoction when it is taken. Or, all the above ingredients can be ground into powder.

Functions: 1. To promote the circulation of *Qi* in the liver. 2. To dispel cold and stop pain.

Indications: Cold type of hernia.

Manifestations:

Lower lateral abdominal pain radiating to the testes ——————— Coldness in the liver channels.

Pale tongue with white coating

Deep and wiry or slow pulse

Explanations:

Signs of *Qi* stagnation in the liver and coldness in the interior.

Herbs and Actions:

Lindera root (Wuyao)

Green tangerine peel (Qingpi)

Costus root (Muxiang)

Areca seed (Binglang)

Sichuan chinaberry (Chuanlianzi)

To promote the circulation of *Qi* in the liver and stop pain.

159

Fennel fruit (Xiaohuixiang) —————————————— To dispel cold and stop pain.

Galanga (Gaoliangjiang)

Croton seed (Badou) —————————————— To relieve the cold property
of Sichuan chinaberry
(Chuanlianzi).

Applications: Hernia and dysmenorrhea.

Modifications: 1. Severe cold. *Add:* Evodia fruit (Wuzhuyu) and Cinnamon bark (Rougui). 2. Dysmenorrhea. *Add:* Ligusticum (Chuanxiong),Carthamus(Honghua)and Chinese angelica (Danggui).

JUHE WAN

—Pills of Tangerine Seed Combination

Tangerine seed (Juhe)	30 g
Seaweed (Haizao)	30 g
Ecklonia (Kunbu)	30 g
Sichuan chinaberry (Chuanlianzi)	30 g
Peach seed (Taoren)	30 g
Magnolia bark (Houpo)	15 g
Clematis stem (Mutong)	15 g
Immature bitter orange (Zhishi)	15 g
Corydalis tuber (Yanhusuo)	15 g
Cinnamon bark (Rougui)	15 g
Costus root (Muxiang)	15 g
Kelp (Haidai)	30 g

Method Used: The ingredients are ground into powder and mixed with wine to make pills, or they can be cooked by decoction.

Functions: 1. To promote *Qi* and stop pain. 2. To soften hardness and remove nodules.

Indications: Testitis or hernia due to cold-damp in the liver channels.

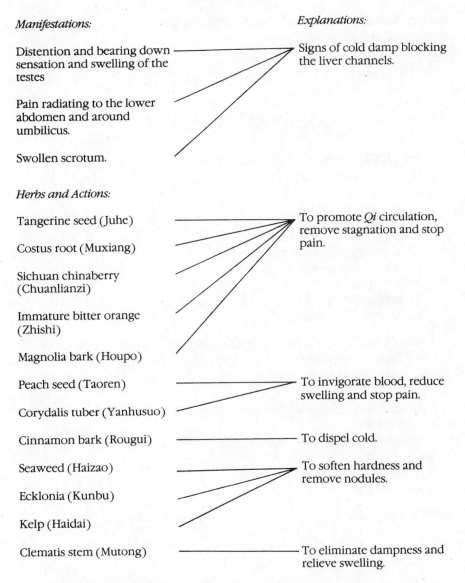

Manifestations:

Distention and bearing down sensation and swelling of the testes

Pain radiating to the lower abdomen and around umbilicus.

Swollen scrotum.

Explanations:

Signs of cold damp blocking the liver channels.

Herbs and Actions:

Tangerine seed (Juhe)

Costus root (Muxiang)

Sichuan chinaberry (Chuanlianzi)

Immature bitter orange (Zhishi)

Magnolia bark (Houpo)

To promote *Qi* circulation, remove stagnation and stop pain.

Peach seed (Taoren)

Corydalis tuber (Yanhusuo)

To invigorate blood, reduce swelling and stop pain.

Cinnamon bark (Rougui)

To dispel cold.

Seaweed (Haizao)

Ecklonia (Kunbu)

Kelp (Haidai)

To soften hardness and remove nodules.

Clematis stem (Mutong)

To eliminate dampness and relieve swelling.

Applications: Epididymitis, testitis and hydrocele testes.

Modifications: 1. Severe cold. *Add:* Fennel fruit (Xiaohuixiang) and Evodia fruit (Wuzhuyu). 2. Prolonged cold-damp transforming into heat. *Replace:* Cinnamon bark (Rougui) with Phellodendron (Huangbai), Scutellaria (Huangqin) and Chinese gentiana (Longdancao). 3. Severe distention and swelling in scrotum. *Add:* Plantain seed (Cheqianzi) and Alisma (Zexie).

SUZI JIANGQI TANG

—Decoction of Perilla Seed Combination to Descend *Qi*

Perilla seed (Suzi)	9 g
Pinellia tuber (Banxia)	9 g
Chinese angelica (Danggui)	6 g
Licorice (Gancao)	6 g
Peucedanum root (Qianhu)	6 g
Magnolia bark (Houpo)	6 g
Cinnamon bark (Rougui)	3 g

Method Used: Two slices of Fresh ginger (Shengjiang), one piece of Jujube (Dazao) and five leaves of Perilla leaf (Zisuye) are added to the mixed herbs listed above, put in water and the mixture is cooked by decoction.

Functions: 1. To descend *Qi* and soothe asthma. 2. To resolve phlegm and stop cough.

Indications: Cough and asthma due to phlegm-fluid blocking in the lungs and deficiency of the kidneys in receiving *Qi*.

Manifestations:

Inspiratory dyspnea

Asthma

Cough with profuse sputum

Stifling sensation in the chest

Shortness of breath

Explanations:

Deficiency of the kidneys caused by their failing to receive *Qi*.

Deficiency of the kidneys caused by their failing to dominate water metabolism; and a part of water turning into phlegm, blocking the lungs; the lungs' function of descending and dispersing impaired.

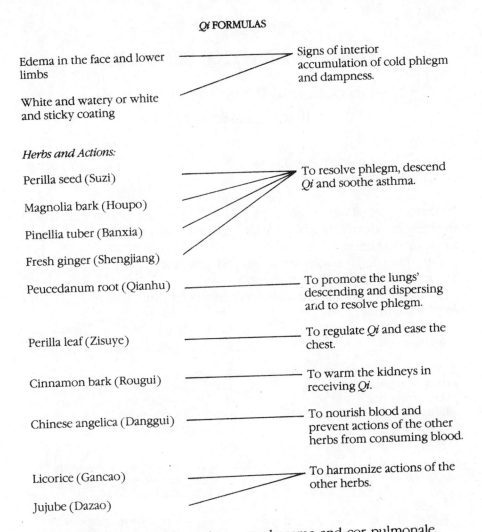

Edema in the face and lower limbs

White and watery or white and sticky coating

Signs of interior accumulation of cold phlegm and dampness.

Herbs and Actions:

Perilla seed (Suzi)

Magnolia bark (Houpo)

Pinellia tuber (Banxia)

Fresh ginger (Shengjiang)

To resolve phlegm, descend *Qi* and soothe asthma.

Peucedanum root (Qianhu) — To promote the lungs' descending and dispersing and to resolve phlegm.

Perilla leaf (Zisuye) — To regulate *Qi* and ease the chest.

Cinnamon bark (Rougui) — To warm the kidneys in receiving *Qi*.

Chinese angelica (Danggui) — To nourish blood and prevent actions of the other herbs from consuming blood.

Licorice (Gancao)

Jujube (Dazao)

To harmonize actions of the other herbs.

Applications: Bronchitis, asthma, emphysema and cor pulmonale.

Modifications: 1. Severe edema. *Add:* Poria (Fuling), White atractylodes (Baizhu) and Alisma (Zexie). 2. Exterior symptoms manifested by chills and fever. *Add:* Ephedra (Mahuang) and Apricot seed (Xingren).

Cautions: 1. The formula is contraindicated in a person with deficiency of the lungs and kidneys, asthma and cough with no sputum. 2. The formula cannot be used with cough and asthma due to heat in the lungs.

TINGLI DAZAO XIEFEI TANG

—Decoction to Purge the Lungs with Lepidium Seed and Jujube

Lepidium seed (Tinglizi)	10 g
Jujube (Dazao)	12 pcs

Method Used: Twelve pieces of Jujube (Dazao) are boiled first, then the Lepidium seed (Tinglizi) is added to the jujube and they are cooked again by decoction.

Functions: 1. To purge the lungs and promote water-metabolism. 2. To descend *Qi* and soothe asthma.

Indications: Asthmatic cough with profuse sputum due to retention of phlegm-fluid.

Manifestations:

Explanations:

Asthmatic cough with profuse sputum

Stifling sensation in the chest that renders lying flat impossible

Lung failing its function in descending and *Qi* in the lungs blocked as phlegm|fluid accumulates in the chest and intercostal region.

Edema of the face, eyes or whole body ———————— Symptom of harmful water or fluid flowing into the skin and muscles.

Scanty urine ———————— Dysfunction of descending and dispersing of the lungs which fail in regulating water passages and promote water metabolism so body fluids cannot be sent to the urinary bladder to be excreted out of the body.

Herbs and Actions:

Lepidium seed (Tinglizi) ———————— To conduct *Qi* downward, promote urination, eliminate phlegm, soothe asthma and stop cough.

164

Jujube (Dazao) ———————————— To promote *Qi* and
strengthen the spleen and
stomach; to prevent the
strong action of Lepidium
seed (Tinglizi) from injuring
the anti-pathogenic factor.

Applications: Chronic bronchitis, cardiac pulmonale and cardiac failure.

Modifications: 1. Severe asthmatic cough with profuse sputum. *Add:* Perilla seed (Suzi), Brassica seed (Baijiezi) and Radish seed (Laifuzi). 2. Yellow sputum, yellow sticky coating or fever. *Add:* Scutellaria (Huangqin), Houttuynia (Yuxingcao) and Trichosanthes (Gualou). 3. Severe edema. *Add:* Poria (Fuling), White atractylodes (Baizhu) and Cinnamon twigs (Guizhi).

DINGCHUAN TANG

—Decoction to Relieve Asthma

Ginkgo seed (Baiguo)	9 g
Ephedra (Mahuang)	9 g
Perilla seed (Suzi)	6 g
Licorice (Gancao)	3 g
Tussilago flower (Kuandonghua)	9 g
Apricot seed (Xingren)	9 g
Mulberry bark (Sangbaipi)	9 g
Scutellaria (Huangqin)	6 g
Pinellia tuber (Banxia)	9 g

Method Used: The herbs are cooked with three glasses of water into two glasses of decoction.

Functions: 1. To promote the lung *Qi* function in descending and dispersing. 2. To resolve phlegm and soothe asthma.

Indications: Asthma due to invasion by exogenous pathogenic cold and existence of heat in the interior.

165

Manifestations: *Explanations:*

Asthma ———————————————— Dysfunction of the lungs in
                                                descending; blockage of
Stifling sensation in the chest ————— turbid phlegm.

Cough with yellow and sticky
sputum

Chills and fever ———————————— Invasion by exogenous
                                                pathogenic wind and cold.

Yellow and sticky coating ——————— Signs of the existence of
                                                heat-phlegm in the interior.
Rolling and rapid pulse ——————

Herbs and Actions:

Ephedra (Mahuang) ————————— To disperse the lung *Qi*,
                                                release the exterior and
                                                soothe asthma.

Ginkgo seed (Baiguo) ———————— To astrict the lung *Qi* and
                                                soothe asthma.

Perilla seed (Suzi) ——————————— To descend *Qi*, resolve
                                                phlegm and soothe asthma.
Apricot seed (Xingren)

Pinellia tuber (Banxia)

Tussilago flower
(Kuandonghua)

Mulberry bark (Sangbaipi)

Scutellaria (Huangqin) ——————— To clear heat.

Licorice (Gancao) ————————— To harmonize actions of the
                                                other herbs.

Applications: Asthma and bronchitis.

Modifications: 1. Severe heat-phlegm. *Add:* Houttuynia (Yuxingcao),
Capejasmine fruit (Zhizi), Trichosanthes (Gualou) and Arisaema with
bile (Dannanxing). 2. Severe stifling sensation in the chest. *Add:* Bitter
orange (Zhiqiao), Citrus peel (Jupi) and Magnolia bark (Houpo). 3.
Severe chills. *Add:* Perilla leaf (Zisuye).

XUANFU DAIZHE TANG

—Decoction of Inula Flower and Hematite Combination

Inula flower (Xuanfuhua)	9 g
Ginseng (Renshen)	6 g
Fresh ginger (Shengjiang)	10 g
Hematite (Daizheshi)	9 g
Licorice (Gancao)	6 g
Pinellia tuber (Banxia)	9 g
Jujube (Dazao)	4 pcs

Method Used: The ingredients are cooked with water by decoction.
Functions: 1. To conduct perversion downward and resolve phlegm.
2. To tonify *Qi* and harmonize the stomach.
Indications: Epigastric fullness, obstruction and belching due to weakness of the stomach and blockage of phlegm.

Manifestations:

Explanations:

Epigastric fullness and obstruction ———————— Weakness of the stomach and blockage of the turbid phlegm.

Belching ———————— Upward perversion of the stomach *Qi.*

Vomiting with saliva

Pale tongue with white and watery coating ———————— Signs of *Qi* deficiency and accumulation of phlegm and dampness in the interior.

Wiry and deficient pulse

Herbs and Actions:

Inula flower (Xuanfuhua) ———————— To descend *Qi* and resolve phlegm.

Hematite (Daizheshi)

Pinellia tuber (Banxia) ———————— To remove stagnation.

Ginseng (Renshen)

Jujube (Dazao)

Fresh ginger (Shengjiang)

Licorice (Gancao)

To tonify *Qi* in the spleen and stomach; to strengthen the spleen and harmonize the stomach.

To harmonize actions of the other herbs.

Applications: Chronic gastritis, gastroptosis, nervous belching or vomiting.

Modifications: 1. Mild *Qi* deficiency. *Delete:* Ginseng (Renshen) and Jujube (Dazao). 2. Cold in the stomach. *Replace:* Fresh ginger (Shengjiang) with Dried ginger (Ganjiang) and Evodia fruit (Wuzhuyu). 3. Heat in the stomach. *Add:* Bamboo leaf (Zhuye) and Loquat leaf (Pipaye). 4. Excessive phlegm fluid. *Add:* Citrus peel (Jupi) and Poria (Fuling).

JUPI ZHURU TANG

—Decoction of Citrus Peel and Bamboo Shavings Combination

Citrus peel (Jupi)	12 g
Bamboo shavings (Zhuru)	12 g
Jujube (Dazao)	5 pcs
Fresh ginger (Shengjiang)	9 g
Licorice (Gancao)	6 g
Ginseng (Renshen)	3 g

Method Used: The ingredients are cooked with water by decoction.

Functions: 1. To conduct perversion downward and stop hiccups. 2. To tonify *Qi* and clear heat.

Indications: Hiccups or vomiting due to weakness of the stomach and existence of heat in the interior.

Manifestations: *Explanations:*

Frequent hiccupping ——————————→ Upward perversion of the
                                  stomach *Qi*.
Nausea ——————————————————————

Vomiting ————————————————————

Red, tender tongue with ————————→ Signs of deficiency and heat
scanty coating   in the interior.

Deficient and rapid pulse ————————

Herbs and Actions:

Citrus peel (Jupi) ——————————————— To regulate *Qi*, strengthen the
                                     stomach and stop vomiting.

Bamboo shavings (Zhuru) ←————————— To clear heat.

Fresh ginger (Shengjiang) ———————— To conduct perversion
                                     downward and stop
                                     vomiting.

                                     To check excessive action of
                                     Bamboo shavings (Zhuru).

Jujube (Dazao) ——————————————————— To strengthen the spleen and
                                     stomach.

Ginseng (Renshen) ———————————————— To tonify *Qi* in the spleen and
                                     stomach.

Licorice (Gancao) ———————————————— To harmonize actions of the
                                     other herbs.

Applications: Vomiting during pregnancy, phrenospasm and incomplete pylorochesis.

Modifications: 1. *Yin* deficiency in the stomach manifested by thirst, dry and little tongue coating, thready and rapid pulse. *Add:* Ophiopogon root (Maimendong), Glehnia (Shashen), Reed root (Lugen) and Loquat leaf (Pipaye). 2. Mild *Qi* deficiency. *Delete:* Ginseng (Renshen).

XI. Blood Formulas

Formulas that regulate blood circulation and treat blood stagnation and bleeding syndromes are called blood formulas. They can be classified into two categories:

1. Formulas for invigorating blood. They invigorate blood circulation and remove blood stagnation and are used to treat syndromes caused by stagnated blood.

2. Formulas for stopping bleeding. They stop bleeding and are used for treating hemorrhagic diseases.

TAOREN CHENGQI TANG

—Decoction of Peach Seed Combination

Peach seed (Taoren)	12 g
Rhubarb (Dahuang)	12 g
Cinnamon twigs (Guizhi)	6 g
Licorice (Gancao)	6 g
Mirabilitum (Mangxiao)	6 g

Method Used: Except for the Mirabilitum (Mangxiao), the other herbs are well cooked in water by decoction, then Mirabilitum (Mangxiao) is added into the decoction for boiling.

Functions: To remove blood stagnation and clear heat.
Indications: Blood stagnation in the lower *jiao*.

Manifestations: *Explanations:*

Spasms, distention and ————————————— Blood stagnation in the lower
fullness in the lower   *jiao*.
abdomen

Increased body temperature ————————— Heat in the Xue (blood)
at night   system.

Thirst   ————————————— Disturbance of the mind; and
                                                     body fluids damaged by heat.

Irritability

Constipation

Deep and excess or choppy ————————— Blood stagnation in the
pulse   interior.

Herbs and Actions:

Peach seed (Taoren)   To invigorate the blood
                                                     circulation and remove
Cinnamon twigs (Guizhi)   stagnation of blood.

Rhubarb (Dahuang)   To drain blood stagnation
                                                     and heat downward.

Mirabilitum (Mangxiao)

Licorice (Gancao)   ————————————— To harmonize actions of the
                                                     other herbs.

Applications: Amenorrhea, dysmenorrhea, acute pelvic inflammation
and placenta retention.

Modifications: Amenorrhea or dysmenorrhea. *Add:* Chinese angelica
(Danggui) and Ligusticum (Chuanxiong).

Cautions: The formula is contraindicated during pregnancy.

XUEFU ZHUYU TANG

—Decoction to Remove Blood Stagnation in the Chest

Peach seed (Taoren)	12 g
Carthamus (Honghua)	9 g
Chinese angelica (Danggui)	9 g
Fresh rehmannia (Shengdihuang)	9 g
Ligusticum (Chuanxiong)	5 g
Red peony (Chishao)	6 g
Achyranthes (Niuxi)	9 g
Platycodon (Jiegeng)	5 g
Bupleurum (Chaihu)	3 g
Bitter orange (Zhiqiao)	6 g
Licorice (Gancao)	3 g

Method Used: The ingredients are cooked with water by decoction.

Functions: 1. To invigorate blood circulation. 2. To promote circulation of *Qi* and stop pain.

Indications: Blood stagnation in the chest.

Manifestations:	*Explanations:*
Stabbing pain in the chest	Blood stagnation in the chest.
Headache	Failure of the ascending of the clear *Yang* caused by obstruction of blood stagnation.
Stifling sensation in the chest	Disturbance of the mind by heat transformed from blood stagnation.
Irritability	
Increased body temperature in the evening	
Insomnia, palpitation	

172

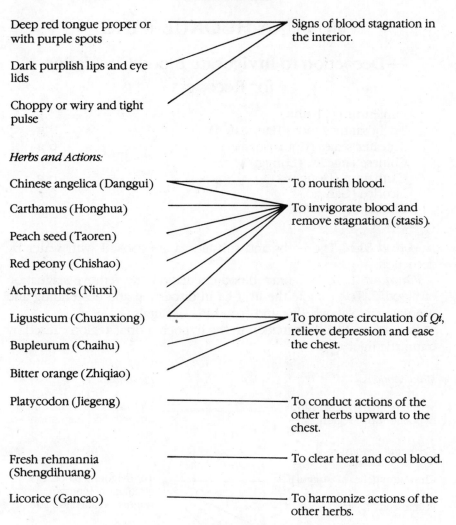

Deep red tongue proper or with purple spots

Dark purplish lips and eye lids

Choppy or wiry and tight pulse

Signs of blood stagnation in the interior.

Herbs and Actions:

Chinese angelica (Danggui) — To nourish blood.

Carthamus (Honghua)

Peach seed (Taoren)

Red peony (Chishao)

Achyranthes (Niuxi)

To invigorate blood and remove stagnation (stasis).

Ligusticum (Chuanxiong)

Bupleurum (Chaihu)

Bitter orange (Zhiqiao)

To promote circulation of *Qi*, relieve depression and ease the chest.

Platycodon (Jiegeng) — To conduct actions of the other herbs upward to the chest.

Fresh rehmannia (Shengdihuang) — To clear heat and cool blood.

Licorice (Gancao) — To harmonize actions of the other herbs.

Applications: Angina pectoris, irregular menstruation and cerebral thrombosis.

Modifications: 1. Amenorrhea. *Replace:* Platycodon (Jiegeng) with Cyperus tuber (Xiangfu), Lindera root (Wuyao) and Motherwort (Yimucao). 2. Blood stagnation in the hypochondriac region. *Add:* Curcuma root (Yujin) and Red sage root (Danshen).

Cautions: The formula is contraindicated during pregnancy.

FUYUAN HUOXUE TANG

—Decoction to Invigorate Blood Circulation for Recovery

Bupleurum (Chaihu)	15 g
Trichosanthes root (Tianhuafen)	9 g
Anteater scales (Chuanshanjia)	6 g
Chinese angelica (Danggui)	9 g
Carthamus (Honghua)	6 g
Licorice (Gancao)	6 g
Rhubarb (Dahuang)	30 g
Peach seed (Taoren)	9 g

Method Used: The herbs and substances are cooked with water by decoction.

Functions: 1. To invigorate blood circulation and remove stagnation of blood. 2. To promote the liver *Qi* in dispersing and descending and promote circulation of *Qi* and blood in collaterals.

Indications: Blood stagnation in the hypochondriac region caused by traumatic injury.

Manifestations:

Explanations:

Severe pain in the chest and —————————— Blockage of liver channels
hypochondriac region   due to blood stagnation.

Herbs and Actions:

Chinese angelica (Danggui)

Peach seed (Taoren)   To invigorate blood
                                             circulation, remove
Carthamus (Honghua)   stagnation and stop pain.

Anteater scales
(Chuanshanjia)

Rhubarb (Dahuang)

Trichosanthes root —————————— To moisten dryness and clear
(Tianhuafen)   heat so as to remove
                                         stagnation.

174

Bupleurum (Chaihu)	———————	To promote the liver *Qi* in dispersing and descending, stop pain and induce the ingredients to extend their actions into the liver.
Licorice (Gancao)	———————	To harmonize actions of the other herbs.

Applications: Traumatic injury, intercostal neuralgia and costal chondritis.

Modifications: 1. Severe pain. *Add:* Mastic (Ruxiang), Myrrh (Moyao) and Ligusticum (Chuanxiong). 2. Severe *Qi* stagnation. *Add:* Cyperus tuber (Xiangfu), Bitter orange (Zhiqiao) and Green tangerine peel (Qingpi).

Cautions: The formula is contraindicated during pregnancy.

QILI SAN

—Powder to Treat Swelling

Dragon's blood (Xuejie)	30 g
Musk (Shexiang)	0.4 g
Carthamus (Honghua)	5 g
Mastic (Ruxiang)	5 g
Myrrh (Moyao)	5 g
Cinnabar (Zhusha)	4 g
Borneol (Bingpian)	0.4 g
Catechu (Ercha)	7.5 g

Method Used: The ingredients are ground into powder. Each dosage consists of 0.22-1.5 grams taken with warm water or yellow wine, or the powder can be mixed with wine for external use.

Functions: 1. To invigorate blood circulation and remove stagnation of blood. 2. To stop pain and bleeding.

Indications: Swelling and pain due to blood stagnation.

Manifestations: *Explanations:*

Swelling and pain of the ———————————— Stagnation of *Qi* and blood.
affected area

Herbs and Actions:

Mastic (Ruxiang)   To promote *Qi* circulation.

Myrrh (Moyao)   To invigorate blood
                                                           circulation, relieve swelling
Carthamus (Honghua)   and stop pain.

Dragon's blood (Xuejie)

Catechu (Ercha)   ———————————— To clear heat, stop bleeding
                                                           and prevent the other
                                                           ingredients from excessive
                                                           invigoration.

Musk (Shexiang)   Aromatic substances to
                                                           promote collateral's
Borneol (Bingpian)   circulation, invigorate blood
                                                           and relieve swelling.

Cinnabar (Zhusha)   ———————————— To promote circulation in the
                                                           blood vessels.

Applications: Traumatic injury, swelling and angina pectoris.
Cautions: The formula is contraindicated for internal use with pregnant woman.

BUYANG HUANWU TANG

—Decoction to Tonify *Yang* and Restore Normal Function of the Five Viscera

Astragalus (Huangqi)	120 g
Chinese angelica (Danggui)	6 g
Red peony (Chishao)	6 g

Earthworm (Dilong)	3 g
Ligusticum (Chuanxiong)	3 g
Carthamus (Honghua)	3 g
Peach seed (Taoren)	3 g

Method Used: The ingredients are cooked with water by decoction.

Functions: 1. To invigorate blood circulation and remove stagnation of blood. 2. To stop pain and bleeding.

Indications: Sequelae of windstroke (apoplexy).

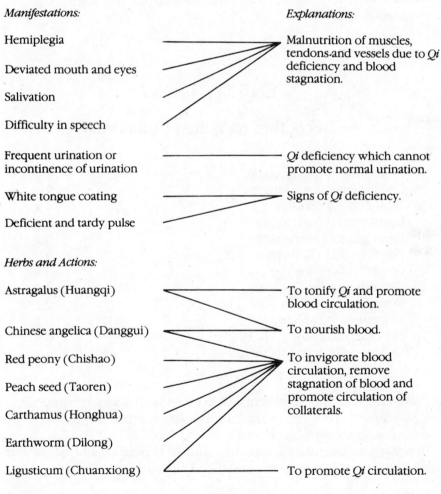

Manifestations:

Hemiplegia

Deviated mouth and eyes

Salivation

Difficulty in speech

Malnutrition of muscles, tendons and vessels due to *Qi* deficiency and blood stagnation.

Frequent urination or incontinence of urination

Qi deficiency which cannot promote normal urination.

White tongue coating

Deficient and tardy pulse

Signs of *Qi* deficiency.

Herbs and Actions:

Astragalus (Huangqi)

To tonify *Qi* and promote blood circulation.

Chinese angelica (Danggui)

To nourish blood.

Red peony (Chishao)

Peach seed (Taoren)

Carthamus (Honghua)

Earthworm (Dilong)

To invigorate blood circulation, remove stagnation of blood and promote circulation of collaterals.

Ligusticum (Chuanxiong)

To promote *Qi* circulation.

Applications: Sequelae of cerebral vascular accident and sequelae of infantile paralysis.

Modifications: 1. Cold limbs. *Add:* Aconite (Fuzi) and Cinnamon twigs (Guizhi). 2. Shortness of breath and lassitude. *Add:* Ginseng (Renshen), White atractylodes (Baizhu) and Poria (Fuling). 3. Profuse sputum. *Add:* Pinellia tuber (Banxia) and Fresh ginger juice (Shengjiangzhi). 4. Difficulty in speech. *Add:* Acorus (Changpu) and Polygala root (Yuanzhi). 5. Dizziness and distention pain in the head. *Add:* Uncaria stem (Gouteng), Chrysanthemum (Juhua), Mulberry leaf (Sangye) and Tribulus fruit (Baijili).

Cautions: The formula is contraindicated in the initial stage of windstroke.

WENJING TANG

—Decoction to Warm Collaterals

Evodia fruit (Wuzhuyu)	9 g
Chinese angelica (Danggui)	9 g
White peony (Baishao)	6 g
Ligusticum (Chuanxiong)	6 g
Fresh ginger (Shengjiang)	6 g
Pinellia tuber (Banxia)	6 g
Ginseng (Renshen)	6 g
Cinnamon twigs (Guizhi)	9 g
Donkey-hide gelatin (Ejiao)	9 g
Moutan bark (Mudanpi)	6 g
Licorice (Gancao)	6 g
Ophiopogon root (Maimendong)	9 g

Method Used: The ingredients are cooked with water by decoction.

Functions: 1. To warm channels and collaterals and dispel cold. 2. To remove stagnation of blood and nourish blood.

Indications: Irregular menstruation due to deficiency and coldness in the Chong and Ren channels and blood stagnation.

BLOOD FORMULAS

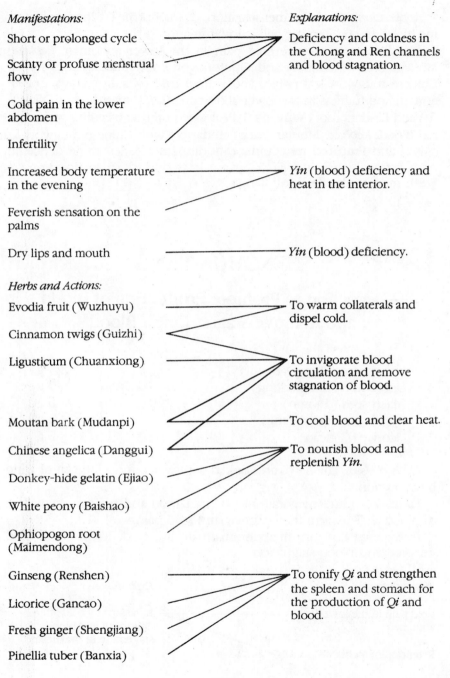

Manifestations:

Short or prolonged cycle

Scanty or profuse menstrual flow

Cold pain in the lower abdomen

Infertility

Increased body temperature in the evening

Feverish sensation on the palms

Dry lips and mouth

Herbs and Actions:

Evodia fruit (Wuzhuyu)

Cinnamon twigs (Guizhi)

Ligusticum (Chuanxiong)

Moutan bark (Mudanpi)

Chinese angelica (Danggui)

Donkey-hide gelatin (Ejiao)

White peony (Baishao)

Ophiopogon root (Maimendong)

Ginseng (Renshen)

Licorice (Gancao)

Fresh ginger (Shengjiang)

Pinellia tuber (Banxia)

Explanations:

Deficiency and coldness in the Chong and Ren channels and blood stagnation.

Yin (blood) deficiency and heat in the interior.

Yin (blood) deficiency.

To warm collaterals and dispel cold.

To invigorate blood circulation and remove stagnation of blood.

To cool blood and clear heat.

To nourish blood and replenish *Yin*.

To tonify *Qi* and strengthen the spleen and stomach for the production of *Qi* and blood.

Applications: Irregular menstruation, dysmenorrhea, functional uterine bleeding and chronic pelvic inflammation.

Modifications: 1. Severe cold pain in the lower abdomen. *Replace:* Moutan bark (Mudanpi) and Ophiopogon root (Maimendong) with Chinese mugwort leaf (Aiye) and Fennel fruit (Xiaohuixiang). 2. Distention and fullness in the lower abdomen. *Add:* Cyperus tuber (Xiangfu) and Lindera root (Wuyao). 3. Prolonged uterine bleeding with light red blood. *Replace:* Moutan bark (Mudanpi) with Chinese mugwort leaf (Aiye) and Prepared rehmannia (Shudihuang). 4. Severe *Qi* deficiency. *Add:* Astragalus (Huangqi). 5. Severe heat due to *Yin* deficiency. *Add:* Fresh rehmannia (Shengdihuang).

SHENGHUA TANG

—Decoction to Promote Production of Blood and Remove Stagnation of Blood

Chinese angelica (Danggui)	25 g
Ligusticum (Chuanxiong)	9 g
Peach seed (Taoren)	6 g
Baked ginger (Paojiang)	2 g
Licorice (Gancao)	2 g

Method Used: The herbs are cooked with water and a little bit of wine by decoction.

Functions: 1. To invigorate blood circulation and remove stagnation of blood. 2. To warm the channels and stop pain.

Indications: Postpartum abdominal pain due to deficient blood, cold invasion and blood stagnation.

Manifestations:	*Explanations:*
Cold pain in the lower abdomen	Invasions by cold after childbirth and blood stagnation in the uterine.
Retention of lochia·	

Herbs and Actions:

Chinese angelica (Danggui)	To nourish blood.
Ligusticum (Chuanxiong)	To invigorate blood circulation, remove stagnation of blood and stop pain.
Peach seed (Taoren)	
Baked ginger (Paojiang)	To dispel cold.
Licorice (Gancao)	To harmonize actions of the other herbs.

Applications: Postpartum inertia of uterus, postpartum metrypercinesia and postpartum retention of placenta.

Modifications: 1. Severe cold. *Add:* Fennel fruit (Xiaohuixiang) and Cinnamon bark (Rougui). 2. Blood stagnation. *Add:* Typhae pollen (Puhuang), Corydalis tuber (Yanhusuo) and Motherwort (Yimucao). 3. Heat transformed from prolonged blood stagnation. *Replace:* Dried ginger (Ganjiang) with Moutan bark (Mudanpi) and Red peony (Chishao). 4. *Qi* deficiency. *Add:* Ginseng (Renshen).

SISHENG WAN

—Pills of Four Fresh Ingredients

Fresh lotus leaf (Shengheye)	9 g
Fresh Chinese mugwort (Sheng'aiye)	9 g
Fresh biota tops (Shengbaiye)	12 g
Fresh rehmannia (Shengdihuang)	15 g

Method Used: The ingredients are ground into powder, then made into pills; or they can be cooked by decoction.

Functions: To cool blood and stop bleeding.

Indications: Spitting blood and epistaxis due to extravasation of heat-blood.

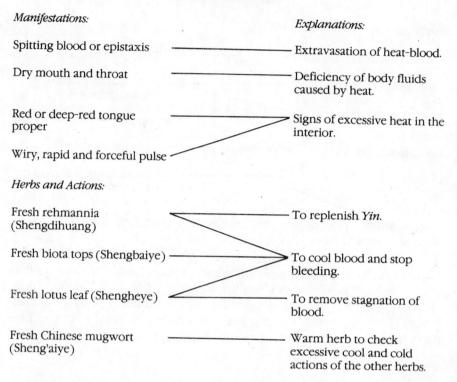

Manifestations:

Explanations:

Spitting blood or epistaxis ——————— Extravasation of heat-blood.

Dry mouth and throat ——————— Deficiency of body fluids caused by heat.

Red or deep-red tongue proper

Wiry, rapid and forceful pulse

Signs of excessive heat in the interior.

Herbs and Actions:

Fresh rehmannia (Shengdihuang)

Fresh biota tops (Shengbaiye) ———————

Fresh lotus leaf (Shengheye)

Fresh Chinese mugwort (Sheng'aiye)

To replenish *Yin.*

To cool blood and stop bleeding.

To remove stagnation of blood.

——————— Warm herb to check excessive cool and cold actions of the other herbs.

Applications: Gastric and duodenal ulcer, bronchiectasis, tuberculosis of the lungs, epistaxis and gingivitis.

Modifications: Profuse bleeding due to excessive heat. *Add:* Coptis (Huanglian), Rhubarb (Dahuang), Madder root (Qiancaogen) and Notoginseng powder (Sanqifen).

KEXUE FANG

—Formula to Relieve Spitting Blood

Natural indigo (Qingdai)   6 g
Trichosanthes (Gualou)   9 g
Capejasmine fruit (Zhizi)   9 g

Chebula fruit (Hezi)	6 g
Costazia bone (Haifushi)	9 g

Method Used: The ingredients are ground into powder, then mixed with honey and Ginger juice (Jiangzhi) and made into pills; or they can be cooked by decoction.

Functions: 1. To clear fire and resolve phlegm. 2. To astringe the lungs and stop cough.

Indications: Cough with blood due to wood-fire impairing metal (lung attacked by liver fire).

Manifestations: *Explanations:*

Cough with bloody sputum ———————— Collaterals of the lung injured by heat.

Red cheek ———————— Excessive fire in the liver.

Irritability ———————— Damage of body fluids by heat.

Thirst

Constipation

Yellow tongue coating ———————— Signs of excessive heat in the interior.

Wiry and rapid pulse

Herbs and Actions:

Natural indigo (Qingdai) ———————— To clear heat, reduce fire and release toxins.

Capejasmine fruit (Zhizi)

Trichosanthes (Gualou) ———————— To clear heat and resolve phlegm.

Costazia bone (Haifushi)

Chebula fruit (Hezi) ———————— To astringe the lungs and stop cough so as to stop bleeding.

Applications: Bronchiectasis and tuberculosis of the lungs.
Modifications: 1. Severe deficiency of *Yin* and blood. *Add:* Ophiopo-

gon root (Maimendong), Glehnia (Shashen) and Trichosanthes root (Tianhuafen). 2. Severe cough. *Add:* Aster root (Ziwan), Tussilago flower (Kuandonghua) and Apricot seed (Xingren). 3. Cough with profuse blood. *Add:* Stemona root (Baibu).

HUAIHUA SAN

—Powder of Sophora Flower Combination

Sophora flower (Huaihua)	12 g
Schizonepeta spike (Jingjiesui)	6 g
Bitter orange (Zhiqiao)	6 g
Biota tops (Cebaiye)	12 g

Method Used: The herbs are cooked with water by decoction, or they are ground into powder.

Functions: To cool blood and stop bleeding.

Indications: Bloody stool due to wind-heat in the large intestine.

Manifestations:

Explanations:

Stool with bright red blood —————————— Injury of collaterals of the stomach and intestines by wind-heat.

Herbs and Actions:

Sophora flower (Huaihua) ——————— To cool blood and stop bleeding.

Biota tops (Cebaiye) ———

Schizonepeta spike (Jingjiesui) —————————— To dispel wind, regulate blood circulation and stop bleeding.

Bitter orange (Zhiqiao) —————————— To regulate *Qi* and ease the intestines so as to have free circulation in the large intestine.

Applications: Hemorrhoids with bleeding.

Modifications: 1. Constipation or sticky stool. *Replace:* Sophora flower (Huaihua) with Sophora fruit (Huaijiao) and Rhubarb (Dahuang). 2. Profuse bleeding. *Add:* Burnet root (Diyu) and Chinese angelica (Danggui). 3. Hemorrhoids and bearing down pain in the anus. *Add:* Red peony (Chishao), Scutellaria (Huangqin) and Chinese angelica (Danggui).

XIAOJI YINZI

—Decoction of Small Thistle Combination

Fresh rehmannia (Shengdihuang)	30 g
Small thistle (Xiaoji)	15 g
Talc (Huashi)	15 g
Clematis stem (Mutong)	9 g
Typhae pollen (Puhuang)	9 g
Lotus node (Oujie)	9 g
Bamboo leaf (Zhuye)	9 g
Chinese angelica (Danggui)	6 g
Capejasmine fruit (Zhizi)	9 g
Licorice (Gancao)	6 g

Method Used: The ingredients are cooked with water by decoction.

Functions: 1. To cool blood and stop bleeding. 2. To promote urination.

Indications: Hematuria.

Manifestations:

Hematuria

Frequent urination

Urgent urination

Scanty urine

Pain in the urinary tract

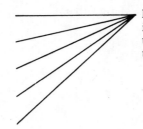

Explanations:

Heat in the lower *jiao* which impairs the *Qi* activity of the urinary bladder and injures the collaterals.

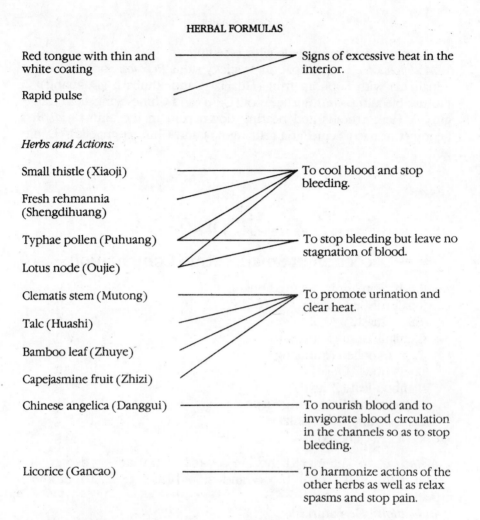

Red tongue with thin and white coating

Rapid pulse

Signs of excessive heat in the interior.

Herbs and Actions:

Small thistle (Xiaoji)

Fresh rehmannia (Shengdihuang)

Typhae pollen (Puhuang)

Lotus node (Oujie)

To cool blood and stop bleeding.

To stop bleeding but leave no stagnation of blood.

Clematis stem (Mutong)

Talc (Huashi)

Bamboo leaf (Zhuye)

Capejasmine fruit (Zhizi)

To promote urination and clear heat.

Chinese angelica (Danggui)

To nourish blood and to invigorate blood circulation in the channels so as to stop bleeding.

Licorice (Gancao)

To harmonize actions of the other herbs as well as relax spasms and stop pain.

Applications: Acute urinary system inflammation.

Modifications: 1. *Qi* deficiency. *Add:* Ginseng (Renshen). 2. Severe pain. *Add:* Amber (Hupo) and Lygodium spores (Haijinsha). 3. Excessive heat. *Add:* Phellodendron (Huangbai).

186

HUANGTU TANG

—Decoction of Ignited Yellow Earth Combination

Ignited yellow earth (Zaoxin Huangtu) 30 g	
Licorice (Gancao)	9 g
Dried rehmannia (Gandihuang)	9 g
White atractylodes (Baizhu)	9 g
Aconite (Fuzi)	9 g
Donkey-hide gelatin (Ejiao)	9 g
Scutellaria (Huangqin)	9 g

Method Used: Ignited yellow earth (Zaoxin Huangtu) is boiled first, then the other ingredients are added to the decoction for further cooking.

Functions: 1. To warm the *Yang* and strengthen the spleen. 2. To nourish blood and stop bleeding.

Indications: Bleeding due to deficiency of the spleen *Yang*.

Manifestations:

Bleeding such as bloody stool, nose bleeding, spitting blood

Dark red blood

Cold limbs

Sallow complexion

Pale tongue with white coating

Deep, thready and forceless pulse

Explanations:

Deficiency of the spleen *Yang* which cannot control the blood.

Blood deficiency.

Signs of deficiency of *Yang Qi*.

Herbs and Actions:

Ignited yellow earth (Zaoxin Huangtu)

To warm the middle *jiao*, dispel cold, astringe and stop bleeding.

187

White atractylodes (Baizhu) ——————

Aconite (Fuzi) ——————

To warm *Yang*, promote *Qi* and strengthen the spleen for controlling the blood.

Dried rehmannia (Gandihuang) ——————

Donkey-hide gelatin (Ejiao) ——————

To nourish blood and prevent the excessive action of White atractylodes (Baizhu) from damaging *Yin* and blood.

Licorice (Gancao) ——————

To stop bleeding.

To harmonize actions of the other herbs

Scutellaria (Huangqin) ——————

To clear heat, stop bleeding and check the strong actions of Aconite (Fuzi) and White atractylodes (Baizhu).

Applications: Functional uterine bleeding and bleeding due to gastric ulceration.

Modifications: 1. Cold manifestations due to *Yang* deficiency. *Add:* Baked ginger (Paojiang) and Chinese mugwort leaf (Aiye). 2. Severe *Qi* deficiency. *Add:* Ginseng (Renshen) and Astragalus (Huangqi). 3. Severe blood deficiency. *Add:* Longan aril (Longyanrou) and Chinese angelica (Danggui). 4. Profuse bleeding. *Add:* Notoginseng powder (Sanqifen), Bletilla tuber powder (Baijifen) and Cuttlefish bone (Wuzeigu).

JIAO AI TANG
—Decoction of Donkey-Hide Gelatin and Chinese Mugwort Leaf Combination

Ligusticum (Chuanxiong)	6 g
Donkey-hide gelatin (Ejiao)	9 g
Chinese mugwort leaf (Aiye)	9 g
Licorice (Gancao)	6 g
Chinese angelica (Danggui)	9 g
White peony (Baishao)	12 g
Dried rehmannia (Gandihuang)	12 g

Method Used: A little wine can be added to the decoction made from the above ingredients.

Functions: 1. To tonify blood and stop bleeding. 2. To regulate menstruation and calm down restlessness of the fetus.

Indications: Deficiency of the Chong and Ren channels which fail in controlling the blood, resulting in such conditions as uterine bleeding, menorrhagia, postpartum bleeding, threatened abortion bleeding or bleeding during pregnancy.

Manifestations:	*Explanations:*
Uterine bleeding	Weakness of the Chong and Ren channels caused by deficiency of blood.
Light red blood without clots	
Pale complexion	
Soreness and weakness of the lower back	Deficiency of blood and essence in the liver and kidneys.
Abdominal pain	Malnutrition of tendons and muscles caused by blood deficiency.
Pale tongue with white coating	Signs of *Qi* and blood deficiency.
Thready and weak pulse	

Herbs and Actions:

Donkey-hide gelatin (Ejiao)	To stop bleeding.
Chinese mugwort leaf (Aiye)	
Licorice (Gancao)	To relax spasms and stop pain.
White peony (Baishao)	To nourish blood, strengthen the Chong and Ren channels and stop bleeding.
Chinese angelica (Danggui)	
Dried rehmannia (Gandihuang)	

Ligusticum (Chuanxiong) ————————— To invigorate blood circulation, promote *Qi* and regulate menstruation so as to prevent bleeding and remove clots.

Applications: Functional uterine bleeding, threatened abortion and postpartum subinvolution of uterus.

Modifications: 1. Severe *Qi* deficiency. *Add:* Ginseng (Renshen) and Astragalus (Huangqi). 2. Severe soreness and pain in the lower back. *Add:* Eucommia bark (Duzhong), Mulberry mistletoe (Sangjisheng) and Dipsacus root (Xuduan).

Cautions: The formula is contraindicated for a person with heat or stagnation of blood.

XII. Formulas for Treating Wind

Formulas that treat all kinds of wind diseases are called treating wind formulas. Wind in Chinese medicine can be exogenous wind, one of six exogenous pathogenic factors or endogenous wind derived from dysfunctions of bowels and viscera, mainly the liver. This group of formulas can be divided into two major categories:

1. Formulas for dispelling exogenous wind. They dispel exogenous wind and release the exterior and are used for treating the exterior syndromes caused by invasion of exogenous pathogenic wind.

2. Formulas for subduing endogenous wind. They are used to treat syndromes caused by a stirring-up of the liver wind due to extreme heat, blood deficiency or *Yin* deficiency.

XIAOFENG SAN

—Powder to Dispel Wind

Chinese angelica (Danggui)	3 g
Fresh rehmannia (Shengdihuang)	3 g
Ledebouriella root (Fangfeng)	3 g
Cicada slough (Chanyi)	3 g

Anemarrhena (Zhimu)	3 g
Flavescent sophora root (Kushen)	3 g
Cannabis seed (Maziren)	3 g
Schizonepeta (Jingjie)	3 g
Atractylodes rhizome (Cangzhu)	3 g
Arctium fruit (Niubangzi)	3 g
Gypsum (Shigao)	3 g
Licorice (Gancao)	1.5 g
Clematis stem (Mutong)	1.5 g

Method Used: The ingredients are cooked with water by decoction, or they are ground into powder.

Functions: 1. To dispel wind and nourish blood. 2. To clear heat and eliminate dampness.

Indications: Rubella and eczema.

Manifestations: *Explanations:*

Skin rash red in color   Skin invaded by exogenous
                                                 pathogenic toxic wind,
Itching of the skin   dampness and heat.

Oozing fluid after rash is
broken

White or yellow tongue   Signs of invasion by
coating   exogenous pathogenic wind
                                                 and heat.
Superficial, rapid and forceful
pulse

Herbs and Actions:

Schizonepeta (Jingjie)   To dispel wind and stop
                                                 itching.
Ledebouriella root
(Fangfeng)

Arctium fruit (Niubangzi)

Cicada slough (Chanyi)

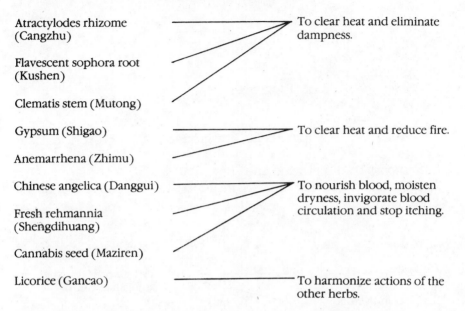

Atractylodes rhizome (Cangzhu)
Flavescent sophora root (Kushen)
Clematis stem (Mutong)
→ To clear heat and eliminate dampness.

Gypsum (Shigao)
Anemarrhena (Zhimu)
→ To clear heat and reduce fire.

Chinese angelica (Danggui)
Fresh rehmannia (Shengdihuang)
Cannabis seed (Maziren)
→ To nourish blood, moisten dryness, invigorate blood circulation and stop itching.

Licorice (Gancao)
→ To harmonize actions of the other herbs.

Applications: Urticaria, rubella, eczema and neurodermatitis.

Modifications: 1. Severe itching due to toxic wind. *Add:* Tribulus fruit (Baijili), Forsythia (Lianqiao) and Lonicera flower (Jinyinhua). 2. Severe heat in the blood. *Add:* Arnebia (Zicao), Moutan bark (Mudanpi) and Red peony (Chishao). 3. Severe damp-heat. *Add:* Broom cypress fruit (Difuzi), Plantain seed (Cheqianzi) and Spirodela (Fuping).

Cautions: When taking the herbs, no hot food, seafood, wine or strong tea should be consumed. Patients should also refrain from smoking.

CHUANXIONG CHA TIAO SAN

—Powder of Ligusticum Combination with Tea

Ligusticum (Chuanxiong)	120 g
Schizonepeta (Jingjie)	120 g

Angelica (Baizhi)	60 g
Notopterygium root (Qianghuo)	60 g
Licorice (Gancao)	60 g
Asarum (Xixin)	30 g
Ledebouriella root (Fangfeng)	45 g
Mentha (Bohe)	240 g

Method Used: The ingredients are ground into powder and taken with tea.

Functions: To dispel wind and stop pain.

Indications: Headache due to invasion by exogenous pathogenic wind.

Manifestations:

Headache

Dizziness and vertigo

Explanations:

Head attacked by exogenous pathogenic wind.

Chills and fever

Nasal obstruction

Exterior invaded by exogenous pathogenic wind which impairs the defensive *Qi*, leading to failure of lung *Qi* in dispersing and descending.

Thin and white tongue coating

Superficial pulse

Signs of the exterior invaded by exogenous pathogenic factors.

Herbs and Actions:

Ligusticum (Chuanxiong)

Angelica (Baizhi)

Notopterygium root (Qianghuo)

To relieve bilateral and vertical headache.

To relieve frontal headache.

To dispel wind and stop pain.

To relieve occipital headache.

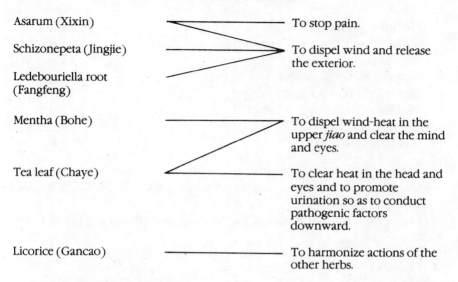

Asarum (Xixin) ———————— To stop pain.

Schizonepeta (Jingjie) ———————— To dispel wind and release the exterior.

Ledebouriella root (Fangfeng)

Mentha (Bohe) ———————— To dispel wind-heat in the upper *jiao* and clear the mind and eyes.

Tea leaf (Chaye) ———————— To clear heat in the head and eyes and to promote urination so as to conduct pathogenic factors downward.

Licorice (Gancao) ———————— To harmonize actions of the other herbs.

Applications: Common cold, influenza, migraine, chronic rhinitis, nasal sinusitis and allergic rhinitis.

Modifications: 1. Wind-heat headache, yellow coating and rapid pulse. *Replace:* Asarum (Xixin) and Notopterygium root (Qianghuo) with Chrysanthemum (Juhua), Chastetree fruit (Manjingzi) and Uncaria stem (Gouteng). 2. Chronic pain. *Add:* White stiff silkworm (Jiangcan), Scorpion (Quanxie), Peach seed (Taoren) and Carthamus (Honghua).

Cautions: The formula is contraindicated in headaches due to *Yin* deficiency or hyperfunction of the liver *Yang*.

ZHENGAN XIFENG TANG

—Decoction to Subdue Endogenous Wind in the Liver

Achyranthes (Niuxi)	30 g
Hematite (Daizheshi)	30 g
Dragon's bone (Longgu)	15 g
Oyster shell (Shengmuli)	15 g

Tortoise plastron (Guiban)	15 g
Oriental wormwood (Yinchen)	6 g
White peony (Baishao)	15 g
Scrophularia (Xuanshen)	15 g
Asparagus root (Tianmendong)	15 g
Sichuan chinaberry (Chuanlianzi)	6 g
Germinated barley (Maiya)	6 g
Licorice (Gancao)	4.5 g

Method Used: The ingredients are cooked with water by decoction.

Functions: 1. To subdue endogenous wind in the liver. 2. To replenish *Yin* and subdue *Yang.*

Indications: Hyperfunction of the liver *Yang* and stirring up of liver wind.

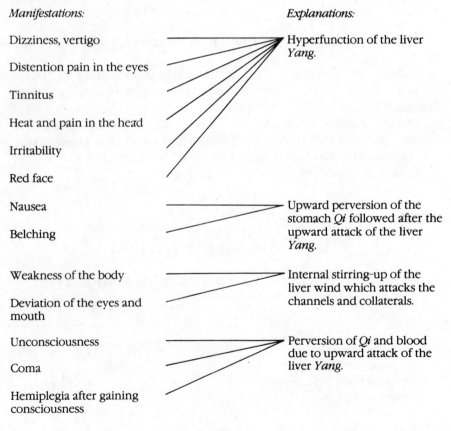

Manifestations:

Dizziness, vertigo

Distention pain in the eyes

Tinnitus

Heat and pain in the head

Irritability

Red face

Nausea

Belching

Weakness of the body

Deviation of the eyes and mouth

Unconsciousness

Coma

Hemiplegia after gaining consciousness

Explanations:

Hyperfunction of the liver *Yang.*

Upward perversion of the stomach *Qi* followed after the upward attack of the liver *Yang.*

Internal stirring-up of the liver wind which attacks the channels and collaterals.

Perversion of *Qi* and blood due to upward attack of the liver *Yang.*

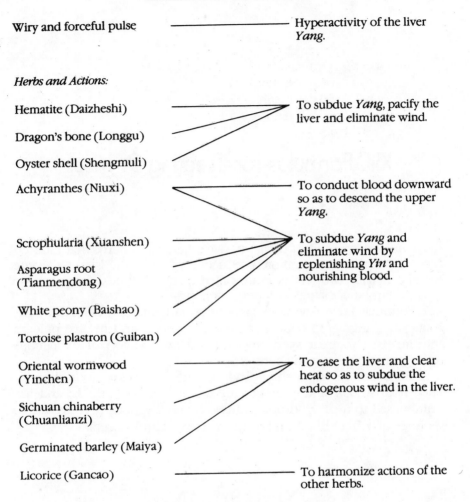

Wiry and forceful pulse ———————— Hyperactivity of the liver *Yang.*

Herbs and Actions:

Hematite (Daizheshi)

Dragon's bone (Longgu)

Oyster shell (Shengmuli)

To subdue *Yang*, pacify the liver and eliminate wind.

Achyranthes (Niuxi)

To conduct blood downward so as to descend the upper *Yang.*

Scrophularia (Xuanshen)

Asparagus root (Tianmendong)

White peony (Baishao)

Tortoise plastron (Guiban)

To subdue *Yang* and eliminate wind by replenishing *Yin* and nourishing blood.

Oriental wormwood (Yinchen)

Sichuan chinaberry (Chuanlianzi)

Germinated barley (Maiya)

To ease the liver and clear heat so as to subdue the endogenous wind in the liver.

Licorice (Gancao) ———————— To harmonize actions of the other herbs.

Applications: Primary hypertension, apoplexy, cerebral hemorrhage.

Modifications: 1. Severe heat manifestations. *Add:* Gypsum (Shigao) and Capejasmine fruit (Zhizi). 2. Severe distention pain in the eyes, nausea and vomiting. *Add:* Prunella spike (Xiakucao) and Sea-ear shell (Shijueming); or Uncaria stem (Gouteng) and Chrysanthemum (Juhua); or Antelope's horn powder (Lingyangfeng). 3. Profuse sputum. *Add:* Arisaema with bile (Dannanxing) and Fritillary bulb (Beimu). 4. Deficient pulse even with heavy press. *Add:* Prepared rehmannia (Shudihuang) and Cornus (Shanzhuyu).

XIII. Formulas for Treating Dryness

Formulas composed of pungent, sweet herbs and herbs that moisten dryness, nourish *Yin*, promote production of body fluids and alleviate syndromes caused by dryness are called treating dryness formulas.

They can be classified into two categories:

1. Formulas for relieving exogenous pathogenic dryness. They invigorate the lungs, stop coughs, moisten the lungs and resolve phlegm and are used to treat syndromes caused by invasion of exogenous pathogenic dryness in the autumn.

2. Formulas for nourishing and moistening endogenous dryness. They nourish *Yin* and promote production of body fluids, and are mainly used to treat syndromes caused by endogenous dryness due to shortage of *Yin* and body fluids in the bowels and viscera.

XING SU SAN

—Powder of Apricot Seed and Perilla Leaf Combination

Perilla leaf (Zisuye)	6 g
Pinellia tuber (Banxia)	6 g
Poria (Fuling)	6 g
Peucedanum root (Qianhu)	6 g
Platycodon (Jiegeng)	6 g

Bitter orange (Zhiqiao)	6 g
Licorice (Gancao)	6 g
Fresh ginger (Shengjiang)	6 g
Citrus peel (Jupi)	6 g
Apricot seed (Xingren)	6 g
Jujube (Dazao)	2 pcs

Method Used: The ingredients are cooked with water by decoction.

Functions: 1. To dispel cool and dryness. 2. To promote the lungs' dispersing and descending and to resolve phlegm.

Indications: Invasion by exogenous pathogenic coolness and dryness.

Manifestations:

Explanations:

Slight headache

Aversion to cold

No sweating

Exterior invaded by exogenous pathogenic coolness and dryness which impair the defensive *Qi*'s function and close the pores.

Cough with diluted sputum

Lungs invaded by exogenous pathogenic coolness and dryness, losing their functions of dispersing and descending with the result that body fluids cannot be distributed.

Nasal obstruction

Sore throat

Lungs affected by exogenous pathogenic coolness and dryness, leading to nose and throat obstruction.

White tongue coating

Wiry pulse

Cold and phlegm-fluid in the interior.

Herbs and Actions:

Perilla leaf (Zisuye)

Peucedanum root (Qianhu)

To dispel cold and release the exterior.

Apricot seed (Xingren)

Platycodon (Jiegeng)

To disperse and descend the lung *Qi*, so as to stop cough.

199

Bitter orange (Zhiqiao) ——————————→ To promote *Qi* circulation,
resolve phlegm and ease the
Citrus peel (Jupi) ————————— chest.

Pinellia tuber (Banxia) ——————————→ To eliminate dampness and
resolve phlegm.
Poria (Fuling) —————————

Fresh ginger (Shengjiang) ——————————→ To regulate Ying (nutrient)
and Wei (defensive) systems.
Jujube (Dazao) —————————

Licorice (Gancao) ————————————————→ To harmonize actions of the
other herbs.

Application: Bronchitis.

Modifications: 1. Severe aversion to cold. *Add:* Allium bulb (Congbai) and Prepared soybean (Dandouchi). 2. Severe headache. *Add:* Ligusticum (Chuanxiong) and Ledebouriella root (Fangfeng). 3. Profuse sputum. *Add:* Aster root (Ziwan) and Fritillary bulb (Beimu). 4. Scanty sputum. *Delete:* Pinellia tuber (Banxia) and Poria (Fuling). 5. Heat manifestations. *Add:* Scutellaria (Huangqin). 6. *Qi* deficiency and weakness of the body. *Add:* Pilose asiabell root (Dangshen).

QINGZAO JIUFEI TANG

—Decoction to Eliminate Dryness in the Lungs

Mulberry leaf (Sangye)	9 g
Gypsum (Shigao)	7.5 g
Ginseng (Renshen)	2 g
Licorice (Gancao)	3 g
Sesame seed (Humaren)	3 g
Donkey-hide gelatin (Ejiao)	2.4 g
Ophiopogon root (Maimendong)	3.6 g
Apricot seed (Xingren)	2 g
Loquat leaf (Pipaye)	3 g

Method Used: The ingredients are well cooked with water by decoction.

Functions: To eliminate dryness and moisten the lungs.

Indications: Damage of *Qi* and *Yin* due to warmth and dryness in the lungs.

Manifestations:	*Explanations:*
Headache	Lungs invaded by exogenous pathogenic dryness and heat which impair the defensive *Qi*'s function and attack the head.
Fever	
Dry cough with no sputum	Injury of *Qi* and *Yin* in the lungs as well as failure of descending of the lung *Qi*.
Asthma	
Dry throat	Damage to body fluids caused by dryness and heat.
Dry nose	
Irritability	
Thirst	
Dry tongue with no coating	Signs of damage to body fluids caused by pathogenic dryness.
Deficient, big and rapid or thready and rapid pulse	

Herbs and Actions:	
Mulberry leaf (Sangye)	To eliminate dryness and heat in the lungs.
Gypsum (Shigao)	To clear heat and conduct fire downward.
Donkey-hide gelatin (Ejiao)	To replenish *Yin* and moisten dryness.
Ophiopogon root (Maimendong)	
Sesame seed (Humaren)	

201

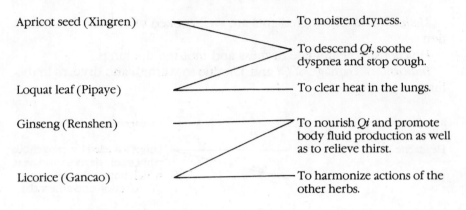

Apricot seed (Xingren) ———————— To moisten dryness.

To descend *Qi*, soothe dyspnea and stop cough.

Loquat leaf (Pipaye) ———————— To clear heat in the lungs.

Ginseng (Renshen) ———————— To nourish *Qi* and promote body fluid production as well as to relieve thirst.

Licorice (Gancao) ———————— To harmonize actions of the other herbs.

Applications: Bronchitis.

Modifications: 1. Cough with sputum. *Add:* Fritillary bulb (Beimu) and Trichosanthes (Gualou). 2. Cough with blood. *Add:* Fresh rehmannia (Shengdihuang) and Biota tops (Cebaiye).

YANGYIN QINGFEI TANG

—Decoction to Nourish *Yin* and Clear Heat in the Lungs

Fresh rehmannia (Shengdihuang)	6 g
Ophiopogon root (Maimendong)	5 g
Licorice (Gancao)	2 g
Scrophularia (Xuanshen)	5 g
Fritillary bulb (Beimu)	3 g
Moutan bark (Mudanpi)	3 g
Mentha (Bohe)	2 g
White peony (Baishao)	3 g

Method Used: The ingredients are cooked with water by decoction.
Functions: To nourish *Yin* and clear heat in the lungs.
Indications: Diphtheria.

Manifestations:

White spots and swollen throat

Sore throat

Dry nose and lips

Cough or no cough

Wheezing

Rapid pulse

Explanations:

Upward attack of toxic heat after invasion by pestilential factors with *Yin* deficiency of the lungs and kidneys.

Yin deficiency and dryness in the lungs which impair the lung *Qi*'s function.

Excessive heat in the interior.

Herbs and Actions:

Scrophularia (Xuanshen)

Ophiopogon root (Maimendong)

White peony (Baishao)

Fresh rehmannia (Shengdihuang)

Moutan bark (Mudanpi)

Mentha (Bohe)

Fritillary bulb (Beimu)

Licorice (Gancao)

To release toxins and relieve sore throat.

To nourish *Yin*, clear heat and moisten dryness.

To cool blood.

To invigorate blood to relieve swelling.

To eliminate dryness and heat in the upper *jiao*.

To moisten the lungs and resolve phlegm.

To clear heat and release toxins.

To harmonize actions of the other herbs.

Applications: Diphtheria, acute laryngitis and tonsillitis.
Modifications: 1. Excessive heat. *Replace:* White peony (Baishao) with

Forsythia (Lianqiao). 2. Severe dryness in the interior. *Add:* Asparagus root (Tianmendong) and Poria (Fuling). 3. Weakness of the body. *Add:* Prepared rehmannia (Shudihuang).

KANG BAIHUO HEJI

—Decoction to Treat Diphtheria

Fresh rehmannia (Shengdihuang)	30 g
Ophiopogon root (Maimendong)	9 g
Scrophularia (Xuanshen)	9 g
Scutellaria (Huangqin)	18 g
Forsythia (Lianqiao)	18 g

Method Used: The ingredients are cooked with water by decoction.
Functions: 1. To nourish *Yin* and moisten dryness. 2. To clear heat and release toxins.
Indications: Diphtheria.

Manifestations:

Explanations:

White spots and swollen throat

Sore throat

— Upward attack of toxic heat after invasion by pestilential factors in summer and *Yin* deficiency of the lungs and kidneys in constitution.

Dry nose and lips

Cough or no cough

Wheezing

— *Yin* deficiency and dryness in the lungs which impair the lung *Qi*'s function.

Rapid pulse

— Excessive heat in the interior.

Herbs and Actions:

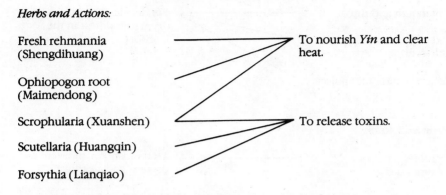

Fresh rehmannia
(Shengdihuang)

Ophiopogon root
(Maimendong)

Scrophularia (Xuanshen)

Scutellaria (Huangqin)

Forsythia (Lianqiao)

To nourish *Yin* and clear heat.

To release toxins.

Applications: Diphtheria, acute laryngitis and tonsillitis.

MAIMENDONG TANG

—Decoction of Ophiopogon Root Combination

Ophiopogon root (Maimendong)	60 g
Pinellia tuber (Banxia)	9 g
Ginseng (Renshen)	6 g
Licorice (Gancao)	4 g
Oryza (Jingmi)	6 g
Jujube (Dazao)	3 pcs

Method Used: The ingredients are well cooked with water by decoction.

Functions: 1. To nourish and strengthen the lungs and stomach. 2. To conduct perversion of *Qi* downward and harmonize the middle *jiao*.

Indications: Consumptive pulmonary disease due to deficient *Yin*.

Manifestations:

Explanations:

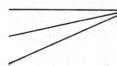

Cough with thin sputum

Dyspnea

Shortness of breath

Deficient *Yin* in the lungs and stomach which leads to upward attack of fire and upward perversion of lung *Qi*.

205

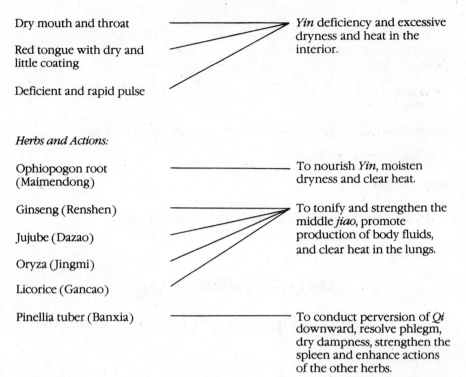

Dry mouth and throat

Red tongue with dry and little coating

Deficient and rapid pulse

Yin deficiency and excessive dryness and heat in the interior.

Herbs and Actions:

Ophiopogon root (Maimendong)

To nourish *Yin*, moisten dryness and clear heat.

Ginseng (Renshen)

Jujube (Dazao)

Oryza (Jingmi)

Licorice (Gancao)

To tonify and strengthen the middle *jiao*, promote production of body fluids, and clear heat in the lungs.

Pinellia tuber (Banxia)

To conduct perversion of *Qi* downward, resolve phlegm, dry dampness, strengthen the spleen and enhance actions of the other herbs.

Applications: Consumptive pulmonary disease due to deficient *Yin*, chronic gastritis and bronchitis.

Modifications: 1. Severe *Yin* deficiency, dryness and heat. *Add:* Glehnia (Shashen), Polygonatum rhizome (Yuzhu), Gypsum (Shigao) and Bamboo leaf (Zhuye). 2. Afternoon fever. *Add:* Stellaria (Yinchaihu) and Wolfberry bark (Digupi). 3. Injury of *Qi* and *Yin* and lingering pathogenic factors in the interior in the late stage of febrile diseases. *Replace:* Jujube (Dazao) with Bamboo leaf (Zhuye) and Gypsum (Shigao).

Cautions: The formula is contraindicated in cold type of consumptive pulmonary disease, but it can be applied to hiccups and vomiting due to *Yin* deficiency in the stomach.

ZENGYE TANG

—Decoction to Increase Body Fluids

Scrophularia (Xuanshen)	30 g
Fresh rehmannia (Shengdihuang)	24 g
Ophiopogon root (Maimendong)	24 g

Method Used: The ingredients are well cooked with water by decoction.

Functions: 1. To nourish *Yin* and clear heat. 2. To moisten dryness and promote bowel movements.

Indications: Constipation due to dryness in the intestines.

Manifestations: *Explanations:*

Constipation ———————————————— Damage of body fluids and
                                                              dryness in the intestines.
Thirst

Red tongue with dry coating ——————— Damage of body fluids,
                                                              dryness and heat in the
Thready and rapid or deep ——————   interior.
and forceful pulse

Herbs and Actions:

Scrophularia (Xuanshen) ———————————— To nourish *Yin*, clear heat,
                                                                      moisten intestines and
Ophiopogon root ——————————   promote bowel movements.
(Maimendong)

Fresh rehmannia
(Shengdihuang)

Applications: All syndromes due to *Yin* deficiency.

Modifications: 1. Excessive dryness and heat in the interior. *Add:* Rhubarb (Dahuang) and Mirabilitum (Mangxiao). 2. *Yin* deficiency and invasion by exogenous pathogenic dryness and heat manifested by sore throat. *Add:* Scutellaria (Huangqin) and Forsythia (Lianqiao). 3. Ying (nutrient) system invaded by exogenous pathogenic heat. *Add:* Rhinoceros horn (Xijiao), Coptis (Huanglian), Lonicera flower (Jinyinhua), Forsythia (Lianqiao), Bamboo leaf (Zhuye) and Red sage root (Danshen).

XIV. Formulas for Dispelling Dampness

Formulas that function to resolve dampness, promote water-metabolism and urination, improve syndromes caused by pathogenic dampness are called dispelling dampness formulas. They can be divided into five categories:

1. Aromatic formulas for resolving dampness. They strengthen the spleen and resolve dampness and are mainly used to treat syndromes caused by dampness blocking the middle *jiao* or disharmony between the spleen and stomach.

2. Formulas for clearing heat and dampness. They clear heat and dampness and are often used to treat syndromes caused by excessive damp-heat.

3. Formulas for removing dampness and promoting urination. They promote urination and are used to treat syndromes caused by retention of water and dampness.

4. Formulas for warming *Yang* and resolving dampness. They warm *Yang*, promote water-metabolism and resolve dampness and are used to treat syndromes caused by retention of water by *Yang* deficiency or cold-dampness.

5. Formulas for dispelling wind and eliminating dampness. They dispel wind, eliminate dampness and promote circulation of channels and collaterals and are used for treating syndromes caused by wind-cold invading channels and collaterals as well as muscles and skin.

HUOXIANG ZHENGQI SAN

—Powder of Agastache Combination to Regulate *Qi*

Areca peel (Dafupi)	30 g
Angelica (Baizhi)	30 g
Perilla leaf (Zisuye)	30 g
Poria (Fuling)	30 g
Pinellia tuber (Banxia)	60 g
White atractylodes (Baizhu)	60 g
Citrus peel (Jupi)	60 g
Magnolia bark (Houpo)	60 g
Platycodon (Jiegeng)	60 g
Agastache (Huoxiang)	90 g
Licorice (Gancao)	75 g

Method Used: The ingredients are ground into powder. Six grams of powder are then added to a soup made of Fresh ginger (Shengjiang) and Jujube (Dazao).

Functions: 1. To release the exterior and resolve dampness. 2. To regulate *Qi* and harmonize the spleen and stomach.

Indications: Invasion by exogenous pathogenic wind and cold; dampness accumulated in the spleen and stomach.

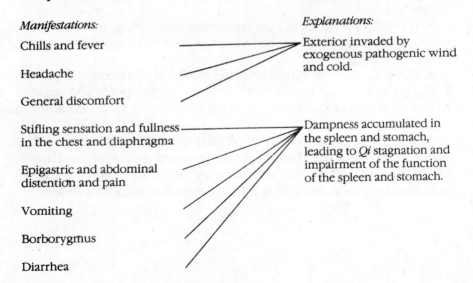

Manifestations:	*Explanations:*
Chills and fever	Exterior invaded by exogenous pathogenic wind and cold.
Headache	
General discomfort	
Stifling sensation and fullness in the chest and diaphragma	Dampness accumulated in the spleen and stomach, leading to *Qi* stagnation and impairment of the function of the spleen and stomach.
Epigastric and abdominal distention and pain	
Vomiting	
Borborygmus	
Diarrhea	

FORMULAS FOR DISPELLING DAMPNESS

No thirst ——————————————→ Excessive dampness in the interior.

Pale tongue with white and sticky coating

Herbs and Actions:

Agastache (Huoxiang) ————————— To stop vomiting.

Perilla leaf (Zisuye) ————————— To release the exterior and resolve dampness.

————————— To regulate *Qi* and ease the chest.

Angelica (Baizhi) ————————— To stop pain.

Magnolia bark (Houpo) ————————— To promote *Qi* circulation, resolve dampness and relieve distention.

Areca peel (Dafupi)

Citrus peel (Jupi)

Platycodon (Jiegeng) ————————— To disperse the lung *Qi* so as to resolve dampness.

Pinellia tuber (Banxia) ————————— To harmonize the stomach and stop vomiting.

Fresh ginger (Shengjiang)

White atractylodes (Baizhu) ————————— To strengthen the spleen and stomach.

Poria (Fuling)

Jujube (Dazao)

Licorice (Gancao) ————————— To harmonize actions of the other herbs.

Applications: Acute gastroenteritis.

Modifications: 1. Indigestion. *Add:* Medicated leaven (Shenqu) and Radish seed (Laifuzi). 2. No chills, fever or headache. *Delete:* Angelica (Baizhi) and Perilla leaf (Zisuye).

Cautions: The formula is contraindicated for a person with yellow and sticky tongue coating or red tongue with little coating.

PINGWEI SAN

—Powder to Neutralize the Stomach

Atractylodes rhizome (Cangzhu)	15 g
Magnolia bark (Houpo)	9 g
Citrus peel (Jupi)	9 g
Licorice (Gancao)	4 g

Method Used: The ingredients are ground into powder. The powder can be taken together with a soup made of Jujube (Dazao) and Fresh ginger (Shengjiang).

Functions: 1. To dry dampness in the spleen. 2. To promote *Qi* and harmonize the stomach.

Indications: Dampness accumulated in the spleen and stomach.

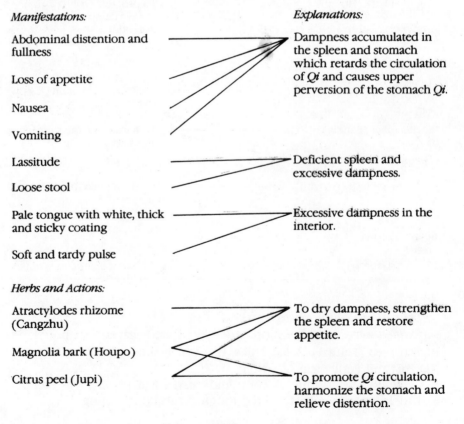

Manifestations:

Abdominal distention and fullness

Loss of appetite

Nausea

Vomiting

Lassitude

Loose stool

Pale tongue with white, thick and sticky coating

Soft and tardy pulse

Explanations:

Dampness accumulated in the spleen and stomach which retards the circulation of *Qi* and causes upper perversion of the stomach *Qi*.

Deficient spleen and excessive dampness.

Excessive dampness in the interior.

Herbs and Actions:

Atractylodes rhizome (Cangzhu)

Magnolia bark (Houpo)

Citrus peel (Jupi)

To dry dampness, strengthen the spleen and restore appetite.

To promote *Qi* circulation, harmonize the stomach and relieve distention.

212

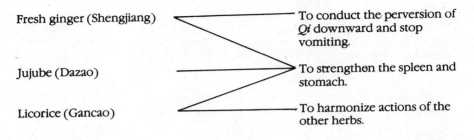

Fresh ginger (Shengjiang) — To conduct the perversion of Qi downward and stop vomiting.

Jujube (Dazao) — To strengthen the spleen and stomach.

Licorice (Gancao) — To harmonize actions of the other herbs.

Applications: Chronic gastritis, gastric and intestinal neurosis and indigestion.

Modifications: 1. Retention of food. *Add:* Medicated leaven (Shenqu), Germinated barley (Maiya) and Hawthorn fruit (Shanzha). 2. Severe abdominal and epigastric distention and fullness. *Add:* Costus root (Muxiang) and Amomum (Sharen). 3. Exterior symptoms such as fever and chills. *Add:* Agastache (Huoxiang), Pinellia tuber (Banxia) and Perilla leaf (Zisuye). 4. Severe diarrhea. *Add:* Poria (Fuling), Plantain seed (Cheqianzi), White atractylodes (Baizhu) and Alisma (Zexie). 5. Cold manifestations such as cold pain in the abdomen, cold limbs, aversion to cold and a desire for warmth. *Add:* Dried ginger (Ganjiang) and Cinnamon bark (Rougui). 6. Heat manifestations such as bitter taste in the mouth, dry throat, yellow and sticky tongue coating. *Add:* Coptis (Huanglian) and Scutellaria (Huangqin). 7. Alternate chills and fever. Add: Bupleurum (Chaihu) and Scutellaria (Huangqin). 8. Constipation. *Add:* Areca seed (Binglang) and Radish seed (Laifuzi).

Cautions: The formula is contraindicated during pregnancy.

YINCHENHAO TANG

—Decoction of Capillaris Combination

Capillaris (Yinchenhao)	30 g
Capejasmine fruit (Zhizi)	15 g
Rhubarb (Dahuang)	9 g

Method Used: The ingredients are cooked with water by decoction.
Functions: 1. To clear heat and dampness. 2. To relieve jaundice.
Indications: Jaundice due to accumulation of dampness and heat.

Manifestations:

Explanations:

Bright yellow color in the
skin and eyes
———————————— Steaming up of the
damp-heat which makes bile
flow out.

Slight fullness in the
abdomen

Thirst

Sweating on the head

Dysuria

Accumulation of damp-heat
which retards *Qi* circulation.

Yellow and sticky tongue
coating

Deep and excess or rolling
and rapid pulse

Excessive damp-heat in the
interior.

Herbs and Actions:

Capillaris (Yinchenhao)
———————————— To clear heat and dampness
and relieve jaundice.

Capejasmine fruit (Zhizi)

Rhubarb (Dahuang)

To promote defecation and
urination so as to clear heat,
fire and dampness.

Applications: Jaundice.

Modifications: 1. Alternate chills and fever. *Add:* Bupleurum (Chaihu)
and Scutellaria (Huangqin). 2. Hypochondriac pain. *Add:* Curcuma root
(Yujin) and Bitter orange (Zhiqiao). 3. Nausea and vomiting. *Add:*
Bamboo shavings (Zhuru) and Loquat leaf (Pipaye). 4. Poor appetite.
Add: Medicated leaven (Shenqu), Germinated barley (Maiya) and Car-
bonized areca seed (Jiaobinglang). 5. Scanty brown urine. *Add:* Talc
(Huashi), Alisma (Zexie) and Lysimachia (Jinqiancao).

GANLU XIAODU DAN

—Dew-Like Pills to Release Toxins

Talc (Huashi)	450 g
Oriental wormwood (Yinchen)	330 g
Scutellaria (Huangqin)	300 g
Acorus (Changpu)	180 g
Fritillary bulb (Beimu)	150 g
Clematis stem (Mutong)	150 g
Agastache (Huoxiang)	120 g
Belamcanda (Shegan)	120 g
Forsythia (Lianqiao)	120 g
Mentha (Bohe)	120 g
Round cardamom seed (Baidoukou)	120 g

Method Used: The ingredients are ground into powder, then mixed with Medicated leaven (Shenqu) to make pills.

Functions: 1. To resolve dampness and turbidity. 2. To clear heat and release toxins.

Indications: Damp-warmth and damp-heat in the *Qi* system.

Manifestations:

Explanations:

Fever

Lassitude

General soreness and weakness

→ Accumulation and steaming up of the damp-heat.

Stifling sensation in the chest

Abdominal distention

Vomiting

Diarrhea

→ Excessive dampness which causes *Qi* stagnation, leading to *Qi* dysfunction of ascending and descending.

Sore throat

Thirst

→ Upward attack of toxic heat.

215

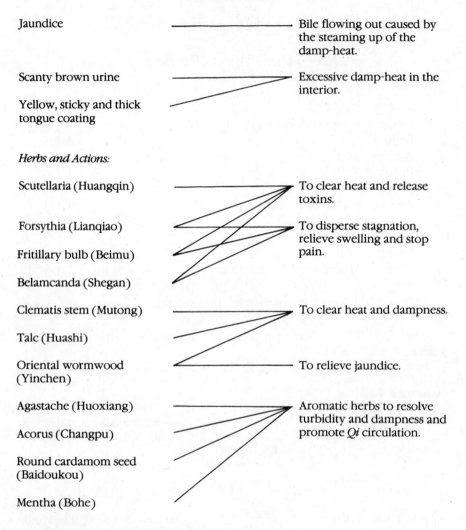

Jaundice —————————— Bile flowing out caused by the steaming up of the damp-heat.

Scanty brown urine

Yellow, sticky and thick tongue coating

Excessive damp-heat in the interior.

Herbs and Actions:

Scutellaria (Huangqin)

Forsythia (Lianqiao)

Fritillary bulb (Beimu)

Belamcanda (Shegan)

To clear heat and release toxins.

To disperse stagnation, relieve swelling and stop pain.

Clematis stem (Mutong)

Talc (Huashi)

Oriental wormwood (Yinchen)

To clear heat and dampness.

To relieve jaundice.

Agastache (Huoxiang)

Acorus (Changpu)

Round cardamom seed (Baidoukou)

Mentha (Bohe)

Aromatic herbs to resolve turbidity and dampness and promote *Qi* circulation.

Applications: Acute infectious icterohepatitis, influenza, biliary tract infection, acute gastroenteritis and typhoid fever.

Modifications: 1. No sore throat. *Delete:* Fritillary bulb (Beimu) and Belamcanda (Shegan). 2. No jaundice. *Replace:* Oriental wormwood (Yinchen) with Bamboo leaf (Zhuye). 3. Abdominal fullness and constipation. *Add:* Capejasmine fruit (Zhizi) and Rhubarb (Dahuang).

216

BAZHENG SAN

—Powder of Eight Ingredients to Clear Heat and Dampness

Plantain seed (Cheqianzi)	500 g
Fringed pink (Qumai)	500 g
Talc (Huashi)	500 g
Capejasmine fruit (Zhizi)	500 g
Licorice (Gancao)	500 g
Clematis stem (Mutong)	500 g
Rhubarb (Dahuang)	500 g
Common knotgrass (Bianxu)	500 g

Method Used: The ingredients are ground into powder, then mixed with water and Rush pith (Dengxincao) for cooking by decoction.

Functions: 1. To clear heat and fire. 2. To promote urination and dispel dampness.

Indications: Urination disturbance due to dampness and heat or urolithiasis.

Manifestations:

Frequent urination

Urgent urination

Painful urination

Scanty and brown urine with the presence of urinary calculi, even anuria

Distention and fullness in the lower abdomen

Constipation

Red tongue with yellow coating

Rapid and excess pulse

Explanations:

Damp-heat in the urinary bladder which impairs *Qi* activity and water passage.

Damage of body fluids by pathogenic heat.

Excessive heat in the interior.

Herbs and Actions:

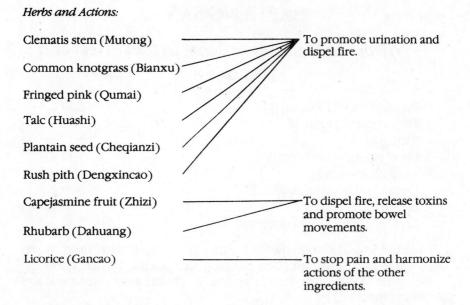

Clematis stem (Mutong)

Common knotgrass (Bianxu)

Fringed pink (Qumai)

Talc (Huashi)

Plantain seed (Cheqianzi)

Rush pith (Dengxincao)

To promote urination and dispel fire.

Capejasmine fruit (Zhizi)

Rhubarb (Dahuang)

To dispel fire, release toxins and promote bowel movements.

Licorice (Gancao)

To stop pain and harmonize actions of the other ingredients.

Applications: Acute urinary infection and urinary system stone.

Modifications: 1. Hematuria. *Add:* Imperata rhizome (Baimaogen), Small thistle (Xiaoji) and Eclipta (Hanliancao). 2. Presence of urinary calculi. *Add:* Lygodium Spores (Haijinsha), Lysimachia (Jinqiancao) and Chicken's gizzard skin (Jineijin). 3. Loose stool. *Delete:* Rhubarb (Dahuang).

Cautions: The formula is contraindicated in person of weak constitution and during pregnancy.

ERMIAO SAN

—Powder of Two Effective Ingredients

Phellodendron (Huangbai)	15 g
Atractylodes rhizome (Cangzhu)	15 g

Method Used: The ingredients are ground into powder.

Functions: To clear heat and dry dampness.
Indications: Flowing downward of damp-heat syndrome.

Manifestations: *Explanations:*

Weakness of the lower limbs ——————————— Flowing downward of
damp-heat.

Pain, swelling and hot
sensation in the knees and
feet

Yellow, thick leukorrhagia

Eczema on the lower part of
the body

Pruritus vulvae

Scanty, yellow urine ——————————— Excessive damp-heat in the
interior.

Yellow, sticky tongue coating

Herbs and Actions:

Phellodendron (Huangbai) ——————————— To clear heat, release toxins
and dry dampness.

To dispel damp-heat in the
lower part of the body.

Atractylodes rhizome ——————————— To dry dampness and
(Cangzhu) strengthen the spleen.

Applications: Acute rheumatic arthritis, vaginitis, vulvitis and inflammation in the lower limbs.

Modifications: 1. Weakness and soreness in the knees and lower back. *Add:* Achyranthes (Niuxi). 2. Pain and swelling in the lower limbs. *Add:* Achyranthes (Niuxi) and Coix seed (Yiyiren). 3. Yellow, thick leukorrhea. *Add:* Euryale seed (Qianshi), Ailanthus bark (Chugen Baipi) and Ginkgo seed (Baiguo). 4. Severe itching and eczema on the lower part of the body. *Add:* Areca seed (Binglang) and Flavescent sophora root (Kushen).

219

WULING SAN

—Powder of Five Ingredients with Poria

Polyporus (Zhuling)	9 g
Alisma (Zexie)	15 g
White atractylodes (Baizhu)	9 g
Poria (Fuling)	9 g
Cinnamon twigs (Guizhi)	6 g

Method Used: The ingredients are ground into powder.

Functions: 1. To promote water metabolism and eliminate dampness.
2. To warm *Yang* and promote production of *Qi*.

Indications: Retention of water and dampness due to deficient spleen and *Qi* dysfunction of the urinary bladder.

Manifestations:

Fever and chills

Headache

Dysuria

Explanations:

Invasion by exogenous pathogenic wind and cold which affect the urinary bladder, obstruct channels and impair the defensive *Qi*.

Thirst

Vomiting immediately after the intake of water

Dysfunction of *Qi* which cannot distribute body fluids and release dampness in the interior.

Pale tongue with white coating

Superficial pulse

Exterior invaded by exogenous pathogenic factors.

Edema

Dysuria

Spleen deficiency which fails in transportation and transformation of water, leading to retention of water and dampness in the interior.

Vomiting

Diarrhea

Deficiency of the spleen and excessive dampness which impair the function of descending and ascending of the middle *jiao.*

Cough

Spitting saliva

Dyspnea

Shortness of breath

Palpitation

Dizziness

Spleen deficiency and retention of phlegm-fluid, in which the phlegm-fluid goes up to attack the heart and lungs.

Accumulation of phlegm-fluid which prevents the clean *Yang* from ascending to the head.

Herbs and Actions:

Alisma (Zexie)

Polyporus (Zhuling)

To promote urination, eliminate dampness, relieve edema and stop diarrhea.

Poria (Fuling)

White atractylodes (Baizhu)

To promote *Qi* circulation, strengthen the spleen and eliminate dampness.

Cinnamon twigs (Guizhi)

To dispel cold, release the exterior, warm *Yang Qi* and promote *Qi* activity in the urinary bladder.

Applications: Edema and acute gastroenteritis.

Modifications: 1. Jaundice. *Add:* Oriental wormwood (Yinchen) and Capejasmine fruit (Zhizi). 2. Vomiting, diarrhea and abdominal distention. *Add:* Atractylodes rhizome (Cangzhu), Magnolia bark (Houpo) and Citrus peel (Jupi). 3. Severe edema. *Add:* Astragalus (Huangqi) and Tetrandra root (Fangji). 4. Severe exterior symptoms. *Add:* Ephedra (Mahuang) and Perilla leaf (Zisuye).

FANGJI HUANGQI TANG

—Decoction of Tetrandra Root and Astragalus Combination

Tetrandra root (Fangji)	12 g
Astragalus (Huangqi)	15 g
Licorice (Gancao)	6 g
White atractylodes (Baizhu)	9 g
Fresh ginger (Shengjiang)	4 slices
Jujube (Dazao)	1 pcs

Method Used: The ingredients are cooked with water by decoction.

Functions: 1. To tonify *Qi* and dispel wind. 2. To strengthen the spleen and promote water-metabolism.

Indications: Accumulation of water or dampness with the exterior invaded by exogenous pathogenic wind.

Manifestations:

Sweating

Aversion to wind

Explanations:

Exterior deficiency due to invasion of exogenous pathogenic wind.

Heavy sensation of the body

Dysuria

Spleen deficiency leading to retention of water and dampness in the interior.

Pale tongue with white coating

Superficial pulse

Exterior invaded by exogenous pathogenic factor.

Herbs and Actions:

Astragalus (Huangqi)

White atractylodes (Baizhu)

Licorice (Gancao)

To tonify *Qi*, strengthen the spleen, consolidate the exterior and eliminate dampness.

To harmonize actions of the other herbs.

Tetrandra root (Fangji) —————————— To dispel wind and promote water-metabolism.

Fresh ginger (Shengjiang) —————————— To regulate the Ying (nutrient) and Wei

Jujube (Dazao) —————————— (defensive) systems.

Applications: Edema.

Modifications: Severe edema. *Replace:* White atractylodes (Baizhu), Fresh ginger (Shengjiang) and Jujube (Dazao) with Poria (Fuling) and Cinnamon twigs (Guizhi).

LING GUI ZHU GAN TANG

—Decoction of Poria, Cinnamon Twigs, White Atractylodes and Licorice

Poria (Fuling)	12 g
Cinnamon twigs (Guizhi)	9 g
White atractylodes (Baizhu)	6 g
Licorice (Gancao)	6 g

Method Used: The ingredients are cooked with water by decoction.

Functions: 1. To warm *Yang* and resolve phlegm-fluid. 2. To strengthen the spleen and eliminate dampness.

Indications: Phlegm-fluid syndrome.

Manifestations: *Explanations:*

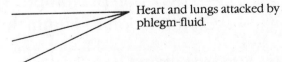

Shortness of breath   Heart and lungs attacked by phlegm-fluid.

Cough

Palpitation

Dizziness   Accumulation of phlegm-fluid which prevents the clear *Yang* from ascending to the head.

Vertigo

Distention ⎯⎯⎯⎯⎯⎯⎯⎯⎯⎯⎯ Retention of phlegm-fluid in
the chest and hypochondriac
Fullness in the chest and ⎯⎯⎯ region.
hypochondriac region

Pale tongue with white, ⎯⎯⎯⎯⎯⎯ Cold phlegm-fluid in the
watery coating interior.

Wiry and rolling or deep and
tight pulse

Herbs and Actions:

Poria (Fuling) ⎯⎯⎯⎯⎯⎯⎯⎯ To tonify *Qi*, strengthen the
spleen, promote urination
White atractylodes (Baizhu) ⎯⎯⎯ and eliminate harmful fluids.

Cinnamon twigs (Guizhi) ⎯⎯⎯⎯⎯ To invigorate *Yang Qi* and
promote water-metabolism.

Licorice (Gancao) ⎯⎯⎯⎯⎯⎯⎯⎯ To harmonize actions of the
other herbs.

Applications: Chronic bronchitis and pulmonary heart disease.
Modifications: 1. Edema. *Add:* Astragalus (Huangqi), Tetrandra root (Fangji) and Alisma (Zexie). 2. Profuse sputum. *Add:* Perilla seed (Suzi), Lepidium seed (Tinglizi) and Jujube (Dazao).

QIANGHUO SHENGSHI TANG

—Decoction of Notopterygium Root Combination to Eliminate Dampness

Notopterygium root (Qianghuo)	6 g
Pubescent angelica root (Duhuo)	6 g
Ligusticum root (Gaoben)	3 g
Ledebouriella root (Fangfeng)	3 g
Licorice (Gancao)	3 g

Ligusticum (Chuanxiong)   3 g
Chastetree fruit (Manjingzi)   2 g

Method Used: The ingredients are cooked with water by decoction.
Functions: To dispel wind and eliminate dampness.
Indications: Exterior invaded by exogenous pathogenic wind and dampness.

Manifestations:	*Explanations:*
Chills	Exterior invaded by exogenous pathogenic wind and dampness, which impair the function of pores and block the channels and collaterals.
Mild fever	
General pain	
Difficulty of motion	
Headache	
Heavy sensation in the head	
White tongue coating	Syndromes of the exterior.
Superficial pulse	

Herbs and Actions:	
Notopterygium root (Qianghuo)	To promote sweating, dispel wind and eliminate dampness.
Pubescent angelica root (Duhuo)	
Ledebouriella root (Fangfeng)	
Chastetree fruit (Manjingzi)	To stop pain.
Ligusticum root (Gaoben)	To invigorate blood circulation and promote *Qi* circulation in the channels and collaterals.
Ligusticum (Chuanxiong)	
Licorice (Gancao)	To harmonize actions of the other herbs.

225

Applications: Rheumatic arthritis and common cold.

Modifications: 1. Wind-cold type of common cold. *Add:* Schizonepeta (Jingjie) and Fresh ginger (Shengjiang). 2. Migraine. *Add:* Bupleurum (Chaihu) and Scutellaria (Huangqin). 3. Headache due to hypertension. *Add:* Pueraria root (Gegen) and Red peony (Chishao). 4. Rheumatic arthritis. *Add:* Large-leaf gentiana (Qinjiao) and Tetrandra root (Fangji).

Cautions: The formula is contraindicated for a person with *Yin* deficiency in constitution: Large dosages are not recommended because they may cause profuse sweating and consume body fluids.

DUHUO JISHENG TANG

—Decoction of Pubescent Angelica Root and Mulberry Mistletoe Combination

Pubescent angelica root (Duhuo)	9 g
Mulberry mistletoe (Sangjisheng)	6 g
Eucommia bark (Duzhong)	6 g
Achyranthes (Niuxi)	6 g
Asarum (Xixin)	6 g
Large-leaf gentiana (Qinjiao)	6 g
Poria (Fuling)	6 g
Cinnamon bark (Rougui)	6 g
Ledebouriella root (Fangfeng)	6 g
Ligusticum (Chuanxiong)	6 g
Ginseng (Renshen)	6 g
Licorice (Gancao)	6 g
Chinese angelica (Danggui)	6 g
White peony (Baishao)	6 g
Dried rehmannia (Gandihuang)	6 g

Method Used: The ingredients are cooked with water into decoction.

Functions: 1. To dispel wind, cold and dampness. 2. To stop pain. 3. To tonify the liver and kidneys. 4. To replenish *Qi* and blood.

Indications: Wind, cold and damp obstructed pain.

FORMULAS FOR DISPELLING DAMPNESS

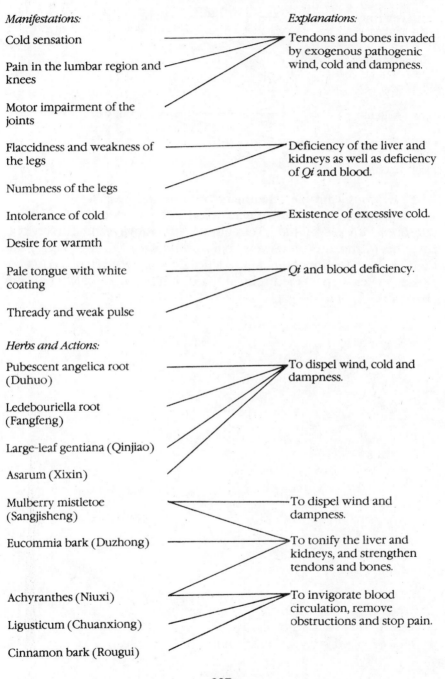

Manifestations:

Cold sensation

Pain in the lumbar region and knees

Motor impairment of the joints

Flaccidness and weakness of the legs

Numbness of the legs

Intolerance of cold

Desire for warmth

Pale tongue with white coating

Thready and weak pulse

Herbs and Actions:

Pubescent angelica root (Duhuo)

Ledebouriella root (Fangfeng)

Large-leaf gentiana (Qinjiao)

Asarum (Xixin)

Mulberry mistletoe (Sangjisheng)

Eucommia bark (Duzhong)

Achyranthes (Niuxi)

Ligusticum (Chuanxiong)

Cinnamon bark (Rougui)

Explanations:

Tendons and bones invaded by exogenous pathogenic wind, cold and dampness.

Deficiency of the liver and kidneys as well as deficiency of *Qi* and blood.

Existence of excessive cold.

Qi and blood deficiency.

To dispel wind, cold and dampness.

To dispel wind and dampness.

To tonify the liver and kidneys, and strengthen tendons and bones.

To invigorate blood circulation, remove obstructions and stop pain.

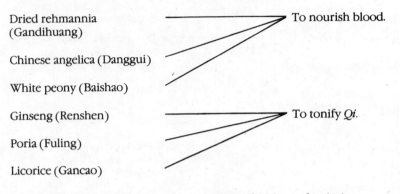

Dried rehmannia
(Gandihuang)

Chinese angelica (Danggui)

White peony (Baishao)

To nourish blood.

Ginseng (Renshen)

Poria (Fuling)

Licorice (Gancao)

To tonify *Qi*.

Applications: Chronic reheumatic arthritis and sciatica.

Modifications: 1. Severe cold invasion. *Add:* Aconite (Fuzi). 2. Severe dampness invasion. *Add:* Tetrandra root (Fangji) and Atractylodes rhizome (Cangzhu). 3. Severe pain. *Add:* Earthworm (Dilong) and Carthamus (Honghua). 4. Mild deficiency of *Qi* and blood. *Delete:* Ginseng (Renshen), Dried rehmannia (Gandihuang) and White peony (Baishao).

XV. Formulas to Expel Phlegm

Formulas that help expel or eliminate phlegm-fluid and deal with syndromes caused by phlegm are called expelling phlegm formulas.

They can be divided into five categories:

1. Formulas for drying dampness and resolving phlegm. They strengthen the spleen and resolve phlegm and are used to treat cough caused by damp-phlegm.

2. Formulas for clearing heat and resolving phlegm. They clear heat and resolve phlegm and are mainly used to treat syndromes caused by heat-phlegm.

3. Formulas for moistening dryness and resolving phlegm. They moisten the lungs and resolve phlegm and are chiefly used to treat cough caused by dryness in the lungs.

4. Formulas for warming and resolving cold-phlegm. They warm the lungs and resolve phlegm and are often used to treat syndromes caused by deficiency of the spleen *Yang* or blockage of phlegm-fluid in the lungs.

5. Formulas for dispelling wind and resolving phlegm. They can dispel exogenous wind and resolve phlegm or dispel endogenous wind and resolve phlegm and are used to treat syndromes caused by wind-phlegm due to the lungs being invaded by exogenous pathogenic wind or retention of turbid phlegm in the interior pulsing that stirs up the liver wind.

ERCHEN TANG

—Decoction of Two Old Ingredients, Citrus Peel and Pinellia Tuber Combination

Pinellia tuber (Banxia)	15 g
Citrus peel (Jupi)	15 g
Poria (Fuling)	9 g
Licorice (Gancao)	5 g
Fresh ginger (Shengjiang)	3 g
Black plum (Wumei)	1 pcs

Method Used: The above ingredients are cooked with water by decoction.

Functions: 1. To dry dampness and resolve phlegm. 2. To regulate *Qi* circulation and harmonize the middle *jiao*.

Indications: Cough due to damp-phlegm.

Manifestations:

Cough with profuse, white sputum

Distention and fullness in the chest and diaphragm

Explanations:

Damp-phlegm blocking the lungs, leading to the lung *Qi* losing its functions of dispersing and descending.

Nausea

Vomiting

Dizziness

Damp-phlegm blocking the middle *jiao* in which the stomach *Qi* cannot descend and the spleen *Yang* cannot ascend.

Palpitation

Heart attacked by the damp-phlegm.

Pale tongue with white, watery coating

Damp-phlegm in the interior.

Rolling pulse

Herbs and Actions:

Citrus peel (Jupi)

To regulate *Qi*, resolve phlegm, harmonize the stomach and stop vomiting.

Pinellia tuber (Banxia) — To conduct perversion of *Qi* downward and stop vomiting.

Poria (Fuling)

Fresh ginger (Shengjiang) — To eliminate dampness, resolve phlegm and strengthen the spleen.

Black plum (Wumei) — To astringe the lungs, stop cough, promote production of body fluids and prevent the other herbs from injuring *Yin*.

Licorice (Gancao) — To harmonize actions of the other herbs.

Applications: Chronic bronchitis and chronic gastritis.

Modifications: 1. Severe dizziness. *Add:* Gastrodia tuber (Tianma). 2. Cold manifestations. *Add:* Dried ginger (Ganjiang) and Asarum (Xixin). 3. Heat manifestations. *Add:* Scutellaria (Huangqin), Houttuynia (Yuxingcao) and Trichosanthes (Gualou). 4. Severe distention and fullness in the chest and diaphragm. *Add:* Bitter orange (Zhiqiao), Perilla stem (Sugeng) and Agastache stem (Huogeng). 5. Indigestion. *Add:* Radish seed (Laifuzi) and Medicated leaven (Shenqu). 6. Insomnia and yellow tongue coating. *Replace:* Black plum (Wumei) with Bitter orange (Zhiqiao) and Bamboo shavings (Zhuru). 7. Severe vomiting. *Add:* Costus root (Muxiang) and Amomum (Sharen). 8. Poor appetite and loose stool. *Replace:* Black plum (Wumei) with Ginseng (Renshen) and White atractylodes (Baizhu). 9. Chills and fever. *Add:* Perilla leaf (Zisuye), Apricot seed (Xingren) and Platycodon (Jiegeng). 10. Red tongue, little and dry coating, dry throat and dry mouth. *Add:* Chinese angelica (Danggui) and Fresh rehmannia (Shengdihuang).

QINGQI HUATAN WAN
—Pills to Clear *Qi* and Resolve Phlegm

Trichosanthes (Gualou)	30 g
Citrus peel (Jupi)	30 g
Scutellaria (Huangqin)	30 g

Apricot seed (Xingren)	30 g
Immature bitter orange (Zhishi)	30 g
Poria (Fuling)	30 g
Arisaema with bile (Dannanxing)	45 g
Pinellia tuber (Banxia)	45 g

Method Used: The ingredients are ground into powder, then mixed with Ginger juice (Jiangzhi) to make pills.

Functions: 1. To clear heat and resolve phlegm. 2. To regulate *Qi* and stop cough.

Indications: Cough due to heat-phlegm.

Manifestations:

Explanations:

Cough with yellow, thick and sticky sputum

Fullness and stifling sensation in the chest and epigastric region

Heat-phlegm blocking the lungs leading to the lung *Qi* failing to control its function of dispersing and descending.

Dyspnea

Nausea

Vomiting

Upper perversion of the lungs and stomach due to *Qi* stagnation.

Red tongue with yellow sticky coating

Rolling and rapid pulse

Heat-phlegm in the interior.

Herbs and Actions:

Scutellaria (Huangqin)

To dispel fire.

Arisaema with bile (Dannanxing)

Trichosanthes (Gualou)

To clear heat, resolve phlegm, ease the chest and remove stagnation.

Immature Bitter orange (Zhishi)

Citrus peel (Jupi)

To soothe *Qi* and resolve phlegm.

Poria (Fuling)	To strengthen the spleen, eliminate dampness and resolve phlegm.
Pinellia tuber (Banxia)	
Fresh ginger (Shengjiang)	To conduct perversion of *Qi* downward and relieve vomiting.
Apricot seed (Xingren)	To soothe dyspnea and stop cough.

Applications: Bronchitis, pneumonia and bronchiectasis.

Modifications: 1. Excessive heat. *Add:* Houttuynia (Yuxingcao), Anemarrhena (Zhimu) and Gypsum (Shigao). 2. Constipation. *Add:* Rhubarb (Dahuang) and Capejasmine fruit (Zhizi).

XIAO XIANXIONG TANG

—Minor Decoction Sinking into the Chest

Coptis (Huanglian)	6 g
Pinellia tuber (Banxia)	12 g
Trichosanthes (Gualou)	30 g

Method Used: The ingredients are cooked with water by decoction.

Functions: 1. To clear heat and resolve phlegm. 2. To ease the chest and remove stagnation.

Indications: Obstruction of heat and phlegm in the chest and epigastric region.

Manifestations:	*Explanations:*
Distention and stifling sensation in the chest and epigastric region, painful if pressed	Obstruction of heat and phlegm in the chest and epigastric region which causes *Qi* stagnation.

233

Cough with yellow and sticky sputum ———————— Upward attack of the lungs and stomach.

Nausea

Vomiting

Yellow and sticky tongue coating ———————— Heat-phlegm in the interior.

Rolling and rapid pulse

Herbs and Actions:

Trichosanthes (Gualou) ———————— To clear heat, resolve phlegm, ease the chest and remove stagnation.

Coptis (Huanglian) ———————— To dispel fire and resolve phlegm.

Pinellia tuber (Banxia) ———————— To conduct fire downward, remove stagnation and relieve fullness and distention.

To resolve phlegm, remove stagnation, descend perversion of *Qi* and stop vomiting.

Applications: Gastritis and bronchitis.
Modifications: 1. Alternate chills and fever. *Add:* Bupleurum (Chaihu) and Scutellaria (Huangqin). 2. Distention and fullness in the chest and epigastric region. *Add:* Immature bitter orange (Zhishi).

BEIMU GUALOU SAN
—Powder of Fritillary Bulb and Trichosanthes Combination

Fritillary bulb (Beimu)	5 g
Trichosanthes (Gualou)	3 g

Trichosanthes root (Tianhuafen)	2.5 g
Poria (Fuling)	2.5 g
Platycodon (Jiegeng)	2.5 g
Citrus peel (Jupi)	2.5 g

Method Used: The ingredients are cooked with water by decoction or ground into powder.

Functions: 1. To moisten the lungs and clear heat. 2. To regulate *Qi* and resolve phlegm.

Indications: Cough due to dryness and heat in the lungs.

Manifestations: *Explanations:*

Cough with little sputum   Dryness and heat in the lungs which cause upward
Difficult to spit out   perversion of the lung *Qi.*

Dry throat   Deficiency of body fluids.

Red tongue with little and dry coating

Herbs and Actions:

Fritillary bulb (Beimu)   To clear heat, moisten dryness and resolve phlegm.
Trichosanthes (Gualou)

Citrus peel (Jupi)   To strengthen the spleen and resolve phlegm.
Poria (Fuling)

Platycodon (Jiegeng)   To promote the lung *Qi*'s function and stop cough.

Trichosanthes root (Tianhuafen)   To promote production of body fluids and moisten dryness.

Applications: Bronchitis.

Modifications: 1. Dry throat and sore throat. *Add:* Scrophularia (Xuanshen), Ophiopogon root (Maimendong) and Licorice (Gancao). 2. Itching in the throat. *Add:* Peucedanum root (Qianhu) and Arctium fruit (Niubangzi). 3. Cough with bloody sputum. *Add:* Donkey-hide gelatin (Ejiao), Fresh rehmannia (Shengdihuang) and Eclipta (Hanliancao).

LING GAN WUWEI JIANG XIN TANG

—Decoction of Poria, Licorice, Schisandra Fruit, Dried Ginger and Asarum

Poria (Fuling)	12 g
Licorice (Gancao)	6 g
Schisandra fruit (Wuweizi)	6 g
Dried ginger (Ganjiang)	9 g
Asarum (Xixin)	6 g

Method Used: The ingredients are cooked with water by decoction.
Functions: To warm the lungs and resolve phlegm-fluid.
Indications: Cough due to cold phlegm-fluid.

Manifestations:

Explanations:

Cough with thin, white sputum

Cold phlegm-fluid in the lungs which impairs the lung *Qi*'s function of dispersing and descending.

Stifling sensation and fullness in the chest and epigastric region

White, watery tongue coating

Cold phlegm-fluid in the interior.

Wiry and rolling pulse

Herbs and Actions:

Poria (Fuling)

To strengthen the spleen and resolve phlegm.

Dried ginger (Ganjiang)

Asarum (Xixin)

To warm and resolve cold phlegm-fluid.

Schisandra fruit (Wuweizi)

To astringe the lungs, stop cough and prevent the other herbs from injuring *Yin.*

Licorice (Gancao)

To harmonize actions of the other herbs.

236

Applications: Chronic bronchitis.

Modifications: 1. Profuse sputum. *Add:* Pinellia tuber (Banxia). 2. Severe cough. *Add:* Apricot seed (Xingren), Aster root (Ziwan) and Tussilago flower (Kuandonghua). 3. Severe stifling sensation and fullness in the chest and epigastric region. *Add:* Bitter orange (Zhiqiao) and Citrus peel (Jupi). 4. *Qi* deficiency. *Add:* Ginseng (Renshen) and White atractylodes (Baizhu). 5. Chills and fever. *Add:* Perilla leaf (Zisuye) and Platycodon (Jiegeng). 6. Dyspnea. *Add:* Ephedra (Mahuang) and Apricot seed (Xingren).

ZHISOU SAN

—Powder to Stop Cough

Platycodon (Jiegeng)	10 g
Schizonepeta (Jingjie)	10 g
Aster root (Ziwan)	10 g
Stemona root (Baibu)	10 g
Swallowwort rhizome (Baiqian)	10 g
Licorice (Gancao)	3 g
Citrus peel (Jupi)	10 g

Method Used: The ingredients are cooked with water into decoction.

Functions: 1. To stop cough and resolve phlegm. 2. To release the exterior and promote the lung *Qi*'s function of dispersing and descending.

Indications: Lungs invaded by exogenous pathogenic wind.

Manifestations:

Cough

Itching in the throat

Slight aversion to wind

Fever

Thin and white tongue coating

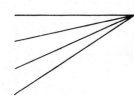

Explanations:

Lungs invaded by exogenous pathogenic wind which impairs the lung *Qi*'s function of descending and weakens the defensive *Qi* in protecting the surface of the body.

The exterior invaded by exogenous pathogenic factor.

Herbs and Actions:

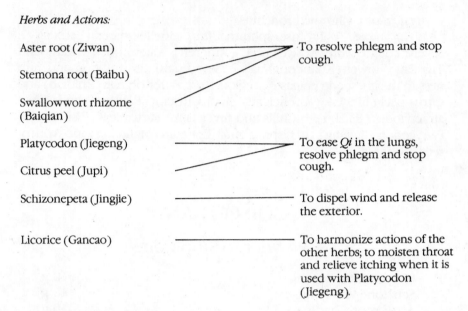

Aster root (Ziwan)

Stemona root (Baibu)

Swallowwort rhizome (Baiqian)

To resolve phlegm and stop cough.

Platycodon (Jiegeng)

Citrus peel (Jupi)

To ease *Qi* in the lungs, resolve phlegm and stop cough.

Schizonepeta (Jingjie)

To dispel wind and release the exterior.

Licorice (Gancao)

To harmonize actions of the other herbs; to moisten throat and relieve itching when it is used with Platycodon (Jiegeng).

Applications: Bronchitis and common cold.

Modifications: 1. Severe aversion to wind and fever. *Add:* Perilla leaf (Zisuye), Ledbouriella root (Fangfeng) and Fresh ginger (Shengjiang). 2. Dry cough or cough with little sputum. *Add:* Fritillary bulb (Beimu), Trichosanthes (Gualou) and Poria (Fuling). 3. Profuse white sputum. *Add:* Pinellia tuber (Banxia) and Poria (Fuling). 4. Profuse yellow sputum. *Add:* Scutellaria (Huangqin), Natural indigo (Qingdai) and Arisaema with bile (Dannanxing).

BANXIA BAIZHU TIANMA TANG

—Decoction of Pinellia Tuber, White Aractylodes and Gastrodia Tuber

Pinellia tuber (Banxia)	9 g
Gastrodia tuber (Tianma)	6 g
Poria (Fuling)	6 g
Citrus peel (Jupi)	6 g

White atractylodes (Baizhu)	15 g
Licorice (Gancao)	4 g

Method Used: The ingredients with a slice of Fresh ginger (Shengjiang) and two pieces of Jujube (Dazao) are cooked with water by decoction.

Functions: 1. To dry dampness and resolve phlegm. 2. To pacify the liver and eliminate wind.

Indications: Dizziness and vertigo due to wind-phlegm.

Manifestations: *Explanations:*

Dizziness and vertigo   Upward attack of wind-phlegm in which wind is produced by liver *Qi* stagnation and phlegm is produced by deficiency of the spleen.

Headache

Stifling sensation in the chest   Upper perversion of the stomach *Qi* due to *Qi* stagnation by phlegm.

Nausea

Vomiting

White, sticky tongue coating   Turbid phlegm in the interior.

Wiry and rolling pulse

Herbs and Actions:

Gastrodia tuber (Tianma)   To pacify the liver and eliminate wind.

Pinellia tuber (Banxia)   To strengthen the spleen, dry dampness and resolve phlegm.

White atractylodes (Baizhu)

Poria (Fuling)

Citrus peel (Jupi)   To regulate *Qi* and resolve phlegm.

Fresh ginger (Shengjiang)   To reinforce the spleen and stomach.

Jujube (Dazao)

Licorice (Gancao)   ——————————— To harmonize actions of the other herbs.

Applications: Meniere's syndrome and neurotic dizziness and vertigo.
Modifications: 1. Severe dizziness and vertigo. *Add:* White stiff silkworm (Jiangcan) and Arisaema with bile (Dannanxing). 2. *Qi* deficiency. *Add:* Ginseng (Renshen) and Astragalus (Huangqi).

XVI. Digestive Formulas

Formulas that aid digestion or remove retention of food are called digestive formulas. The indigestion or retention of food may be due to irregular food intake, liver *Qi* stagnation, or weakness of the spleen and stomach in transformation and transportation.

Since the prolonged accumulation of food may transform into heat or cold, it is not enough to use the digestive formula alone. The digestive formula should be combined with either herbs for regulating *Qi* or herbs for dispelling cold or heat. In a word, selection of herbs mainly depends upon the syndrome—whether it is cold, heat, deficiency or excess.

As to their properties, some digestive formulas are hot in nature, some cold in nature, some function to dispel pathogenic factors and some lessen deficiencies and strengthen anti-pathogenic factors (body resistance).

BAOHE WAN

—Pills to Keep the Function of the Stomach in Good Condition

Hawthorn fruit (Shanzha)	180 g
Medicated leaven (Shenqu)	60 g
Pinellia tuber (Banxia)	90 g

Poria (Fuling)	90 g
Citrus peel (Jupi)	30 g
Forsythia (Lianqiao)	30 g
Turnip seed (Luobozi)	30 g

Method Used: The ingredients are ground into powder, then mixed with water to make pills.

Functions: To promote digestion and harmonize the stomach.

Indications: Retention of food and indigestion due to irregular food intake.

Manifestations:

Distention and fullness in the epigastric and abdominal regions

Belching

Acid regurgitation

Nausea

Vomiting

Poor appetite

Irregular bowel movements

Rolling pulse

Sticky tongue coating

Explanations:

Upward perversion of the stomach *Qi* and heat due to *Qi* stagnation by retention of food in the stomach.

Disharmony of the stomach *Qi.*

Impairment of intestines in transportation.

Retention of food in the interior.

Herbs and Actions:

Hawthorn fruit (Shanzha)

Medicated leaven (Shenqu)

Turnip seed (Luobozi)

To aid digestion.

To descend *Qi* downward and relieve distention.

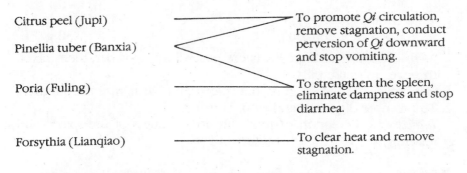

Citrus peel (Jupi) ——————— To promote *Qi* circulation, remove stagnation, conduct perversion of *Qi* downward and stop vomiting.

Pinellia tuber (Banxia)

Poria (Fuling) ——————— To strengthen the spleen, eliminate dampness and stop diarrhea.

Forsythia (Lianqiao) ——————— To clear heat and remove stagnation.

Applications: Indigestion and gastroenteritis.

Modifications: 1. Severe vomiting, diarrhea, fever or dysentery with retention of food. *Add:* Coptis (Huanglian), Scutellaria (Huangqin) and Pueraria root (Gegen). 2. Severe abdominal distention. *Add:* Costus root (Muxiang), Immature bitter orange (Zhishi) and Magnolia bark (Houpo). 3. Constipation. *Add:* Rhubarb (Dahuang) and Areca seed (Binglang). 4. Disharmony of the liver and stomach manifested by distention and fullness in the chest and hypochondriac regions, irritability and hot temper. *Add:* Bupleurum (Chaihu), Curcuma root (Yujin), Cyperus tuber (Xiangfu) and White peony (Baishao).

JIANPI WAN

—Pills to Strengthen the Spleen

White atractylodes (Baizhu)	75 g
Costus root (Muxiang)	22 g
Coptis (Huanglian)	22 g
Licorice (Gancao)	22 g
Poria (Fuling)	60 g
Ginseng (Renshen)	45 g
Medicated leaven (Shenqu)	30 g
Citrus peel (Jupi)	30 g
Amomum (Sharen)	39 g
Germinated barley (Maiya)	30 g
Hawthorn fruit (Shanzha)	30 g

Dioscorea (Shanyao)	30 g
Nutmeg (Roudoukou)	30 g

Method Used: The ingredients are ground into powder, then mixed with water to make pills.

Functions: 1. To strengthen the spleen and harmonize the stomach. 2. To promote digestion and stop diarrhea.

Indications: Retention of food due to weakness of the spleen and stomach.

Manifestations: *Explanations:*

Poor appetite ————————————— Weakness of the spleen and
                                              stomach which fails in
Retention of food —————————— digestion.

Fullness in the epigastric and ——————— *Qi* stagnation caused by
abdominal regions   retention of food.

Loose stool ————————————— Weakness of the spleen in
                                              transportation and
                                              transformation of water.

Sticky and slightly yellow ——————— Weakness of anti-pathogenic
tongue coating   factor, retention of food and
                                              presence of heat caused by
Deficient and weak pulse ——————— retention.

Herbs and Actions:

Ginseng (Renshen) —————————— To tonify *Qi* in the middle
                                              jiao and strengthen the
White atractylodes (Baizhu) —————— spleen and stomach.

Poria (Fuling)

Licorice (Gancao)

Dioscorea (Shanyao) ————————— To strengthen the spleen and
                                              stop diarrhea.
Nutmeg (Roudoukou)

Hawthorn fruit (Shanzha) —————— To promote digestion.

Medicated leaven (Shenqu)

Germinated barley (Maiya)

Costus root (Muxiang) ——————————— To promote *Qi* circulation,
relieve distention and restore
Amomum (Sharen) ——————————— appetite.

Citrus peel (Jupi)

Coptis (Huanglian) ——————————— To clear heat and dry
dampness.

Applications: Gastroenteritis and indigestion.

Modifications: 1. No heat manifestations. *Delete:* Coptis (Huanglian). 2. Deficiency and coldness in the middle *jiao*. *Replace:* Coptis (Huanglian) with Fresh ginger (Shengjiang), and add Aconite (Fuzi) and Evodia fruit (Wuzhuyu).

ZHI SHU WAN

—Pills of Immature Bitter Orange and White Atractylodes

Immature bitter orange (Zhishi)   30 g
White atractylodes (Baizhu)   60 g

Method Used: The ingredients are ground into powder and made into pills. Take 6-9 grams of pills with rice soup or lotus leaf soup.

Functions: 1. To strengthen the spleen. 2. To relieve fullness.

Indications: Retention of food due to weakness of the spleen and stomach.

Manifestations: *Explanations:*

Abdominal distention and ——————————— *Qi* stagnation and retention
fullness   of food due to weakness of
                                                     the spleen and stomach.
Poor appetite

White tongue coating ——————————— Deficiency of *Qi* of the spleen
                                                     and stomach or deficiency of
Deficient pulse   anti-pathogenic factors.

245

Herbs and Actions:

Immature bitter orange (Zhishi)	To descend *Qi*, remove stagnation and relieve fullness.
Lotus leaf (Heye)	To help *Qi* of the spleen and stomach perform their normal functions of ascending and descending.
White atractylodes (Baizhu)	To dry dampness and strengthen transportation.
Rice soup (Miyin)	To tonify *Qi* in the spleen and stomach.

Applications: Chronic gastritis and gastroptosis.

Modifications: 1. Severe *Qi* deficiency. *Add:* Ginseng (Renshen) and Poria (Fuling). 2. Severe indigestion. *Add:* Medicated leaven (Shenqu), Hawthorn fruit (Shanzha) and Germinated barley (Maiya). 3. Severe abdominal and epigastric distention and fullness. *Add:* Costus root (Muxiang) and Amomum (Sharen).

MUXIANG BINGLANG WAN

—Pills of Costus Root and Areca Seed Combination

Costus root (Muxiang)	30 g
Areca seed (Binglang)	30 g
Green tangerine peel (Qingpi)	30 g
Citrus peel (Jupi)	30 g
Zedoary (Ezhu)	30 g
Coptis (Huanglian)	30 g
Phellodendron (Huangbai)	30 g
Rhubarb (Dahuang)	15 g
Cyperus tuber (Xiangfu)	60 g
Pharbitis seed (Qianniuzi)	60 g

Method Used: The ingredients are ground into powder and made into pills.

Functions: 1. To promote *Qi* circulation and remove stagnation. 2. To clear heat.

Indications: Constipation or dysentery due to accumulation of damp-heat in the interior.

Manifestations:

Explanations:

Fullness, distention and pain in the epigastric region and abdomen ——————— *Qi* stagnation due to accumulation of dampness.

Constipation

Dysentery

Tenesmus

Impairment of the intestines in transportation by *Qi* stagnation due to accumulation of damp-heat.

Pus-like and bloody stool ——————— Blood vessels damaged by damp-heat.

Yellow, sticky tongue coating ——————— Accumulation of damp-heat in the interior.

Excess and forceful pulse

Herbs and Actions:

Costus root (Muxiang)

Areca seed (Binglang)

To promote *Qi* circulation and remove stagnation.

Rhubarb (Dahuang)

Pharbitis seed (Qianniuzi)

To promote bowel movements and clear heat.

Green tangerine peel (Qingpi)

Citrus peel (Jupi)

Cyperus tuber (Xiangfu)

Zedoary (Ezhu)

To promote *Qi* circulation and eliminate accumulation.

Phellodendron (Huangbai)

Coptis (Huanglian)

To clear heat, dry dampness
and relieve dysentery.

Applications: Dysentery.

Modifications: Dysentery due to damp-heat. *Replace:* Citrus peel (Jupi), Zedoary (Ezhu) and Pharbitis seed (Qianniuzi) with Pulsatilla root (Baitouweng) and White peony (Baishao).

Cautions: The formula is contraindicated in cases of severe deficiency of anti-pathogenic factors.

XVII. Formulas for Dispelling Parasitic Worms

Formulas that can dispel parasites in the human body are called dispelling parasitic worm formulas. According to the different types of parasitic worms and different natures of syndromes like deficient, excess, cold and heat syndromes, the formulas can be used in combination with the corresponding herbs. Generally speaking, the dispelling parasitic worm formulas are often combined with draining formulas to discharge worms out of the body. These types of formulas are toxic; they should be used with caution for a weak or aged patient, or a pregnant woman. The decoctions or pills are most effective when taken before meals.

WUMEI WAN

—Pills of Black Plum Combination

Black plum (Wumei)	480 g
Asarum (Xixin)	180 g
Dried ginger (Ganjiang)	300 g
Coptis (Huanglian)	480 g
Chinese angelica (Danggui)	120 g
Aconite (Fuzi)	180 g

Zanthoxylum (Shujiao)	120 g
Cinnamon twigs (Guizhi)	180 g
Ginseng (Renshen)	180 g
Phellodendron (Huangbai)	180 g

Method Used: Black plum (Wumei) is soaked in vinegar overnight, then mixed with the powder of the other ingredients and honey to make pills.

Functions: 1. To warm the internal viscera. 2. To dispel the parasites.

Indications: Cold limbs due to ascariasis, and dysentery.

Manifestations:

Explanations:

Abdominal pain

Irritability

Vomiting

Coldness in the intestines, heat in the stomach and restless ascaris in the interior.

Cold limbs —————— Imbalance of *Yin* and *Yang*.

Intermittent abdominal pain ———— Restless ascaris.

Chronic diarrhea

Chronic dysentery

Weakness of anti-pathogenic factors, existence of cold complicated with heat and impairment of transportation of the intestines.

Herbs and Actions:

Black plum (Wumei) —————— Sour herb to calm ascaris and astringe intestines for relieving dysentery.

Asarum (Xixin)

Zanthoxylum (Shujiao)

Cinnamon twigs (Guizhi)

Aconite (Fuzi)

Pungent and hot herbs to calm ascaris and dispel cold.

Coptis (Huanglian)

Phellodendron (Huangbai)

Bitter and cold herbs to drain ascaris downward and clear heat for relieving dysentery.

Ginseng (Renshen) ———————————→ To tonify *Qi* and nourish
blood for treating deficiency
Chinese angelica (Danggui) ———————— syndromes.

Applications: Biliary ascariasis, chronic enteritis and chronic dysentery.
Modifications: 1. Severe coldness in the interior. *Delete:* Phellodendron
(Huangbai). 2. Slight coldness in the interior. *Delete:* Cinnamon twigs
(Guizhi) and Aconite (Fuzi). 3. Normal functions of anti-pathogenic
factors. *Delete:* Ginseng (Renshen) and Chinese angelica (Danggui). 4.
Severe abdominal pain. *Add:* Costus root (Muxiang) and Sichuan chinaberry (Chuanlianzi). 5. To increase the effect of dispelling ascaris. *Add:*
Rhubarb (Dahuang) and Areca seed (Binglang).

QUTAO TANG

—Tapeworm-Expelling Decoction

Pumpkin seed (Nanguazi)   60-120 g
Areca seed (Binglang)   30-60 g

Method Used: The decoction should be taken before meals, preferably
early in the morning. Pumpkin seed (Nanguazi) is chewed first; after
two hours the decoction of Areca seed (Binglang) can be taken. The
tapeworm will be expelled through defecation about four hours later.
In case there is no defecation, Dried Glauber's salt (Xuanmingfen) can
be taken with water to aid bowel movements.
Functions: To expel tapeworm.
Indications: Cestodiasis.

Manifestations: *Explanations:*

Abdominal pain ————————————— Tapeworm stirring in the
interior.
Indigestion ————————————

White proglottids in the stool ————————— Tapeworm in the interior.

Herbs and Actions:

Pumpkin seed (Nanguazi) ————————⟶ To kill tapeworm.

Areca seed (Binglang) ————————⟶ To promote bowel movements and expel tapeworm.

Cautions: The dosage of the decoction for an old, weak person, child or pregnant woman should be limited according to the doctor's advice.

Appendix

A LIST OF APPLICABLE CHINESE HERBAL MEDICINE

Achyranthes (Niuxi　牛夕)

Aconite (Fuzi　附子)

Acorus (Changpu　菖蒲)

Agastache (Huoxiang　藿香)

Agastache stem (Huogeng　藿梗)

Ailanthus bark (Chugen Baipi　樗根白皮)

Alisma (Zexie　泽泻)

Allium bulb (Congbai　葱白)

Amber (Hupo　琥珀)

American ginseng (Xiyangshen　西洋参)

Amomum (Sharen　砂仁)

Anemarrhena (Zhimu　知母)

Angelica (Baizhi　白芷)

Anteater scales (Chuanshanjia　穿山甲)

Antelope's horn (Lingyangjiao　羚羊角)

Antelope's horn powder (Ling-yangfen　羚羊粉)

Antler gelatin (Lujiaojiao　鹿角胶)

Apricot seed (Xingren　杏仁)

Arctium fruit (Niubangzi　牛蒡子)

Areca peel (Dafupi　大腹皮)

Areca seed (Binglang　槟榔)

Arisaema with bile (Dannanxing　胆南星)

Arnebia (Zicao　紫草)

Asarum (Xixin　细辛)

Asparagus root (Tianmendong　天门冬)

Aster root (Ziwan　紫菀)

Astragalus (Huangqi　黄芪)

Atractylodes rhizome (Cangzhu　苍术)

Baked coix seed (Chaoyiren　炒薏仁)

Baked ginger (Paojiang　炮姜)

Baked licorice (Zhigancao 炙甘草)

Bamboo juice (Zhuli 竹沥)

Bamboo leaf (Zhuye 竹叶)

Bamboo shavings (Zhuru 竹茹)

Belamcanda (Shegan 射干)

Benincasa seed (Dongguazi 冬瓜子)

Biota seed (Baiziren 柏子仁)

Biota tops (Cebaiye 侧柏叶)

Bitter orange (Zhiqiao 枳壳)

Black plum (Wumei 乌梅)

Bletilla tuber powder (Baijifen 白芨粉)

Borneol (Bingpian 冰片)

Bos calculus (Niuhuang 牛黄)

Brassica seed (Baijiezi 白芥子)

Broom cypress fruit (Difuzi 地肤子)

Bupleurum (Chaihu 柴胡)

Burnet root (Diyu 地榆)

Caesalpinia (Shilianzi 石莲子)

Cannabis seed (Maziren 麻子仁)

Capejasmine fruit (Zhizi 栀子)

Capillaris (Yinchenhao 茵陈蒿)

Carbonized areca seed (Jiaobin-lang 焦槟榔)

Carbonized petiole (Zonglütan 棕榈炭)

Carthamus (Honghua 红花)

Cassia (Juemingzi 决明子)

Catechu (Ercha 儿茶)

Chastetree fruit (Manjingzi 蔓荆子)

Chebula fruit (Hezi 诃子)

Chicken's gizzard skin (Jineijin 鸡内金)

Chinese angelica (Danggui 当归)

Chinese gentiana (Longdancao 龙胆草)

Chinese mugwort leaf (Aiye 艾叶)

Chrysanthemum (Juhua 菊花)

Cicada slough (Chanyi 蝉衣)

Cimicifuga (Shengma 升麻)

Cinnamon bark (Rougui 肉桂)

Cinnamon twigs (Guizhi 桂枝)

Cinnabar (Zhusha 朱砂)

Cistanche (Roucongrong 肉苁蓉)

Citron (Xiangyuan 香橼)

Citrus peel (Jupi 橘皮)

Clematis stem (Mutong 木通)

Cloves (Dingxiang 丁香)

Coix seed (Yiyiren 薏苡仁)

Common knotgrass (Bianxu 萹蓄)

Coptis (Huanglian 黄连)

Cornus (Shanzhuyu 山茱萸)

Corydalis tuber (Yanhusuo 延胡索)

Costazia bone (Haifushi 海浮石)

Costus root (Muxiang 木香)

Croton seed (Badou 巴豆)

Curcuma root (Yujin 郁金)

Cuttlefish bone (Wuzeigu 乌贼骨)

Cynomorium (Suoyang 锁阳)

Cyperus tuber (Xiangfu 香附)

Dandelion (Pugongying 蒲公英)

Deglued antler powder (Lujiao-shuang 鹿角霜)

Dendrobium (Shihu 石斛)

Dichroa root (Changshan 常山)

Dioscorea (Shanyao 山药)

Dipsacus root (Xuduan 续断)

Dodder seed (Tusizi 菟丝子)

Dogwood fruit (Shanyurou 山萸肉)

Dolichos seed (Biandou 扁豆)

Donkey-hide gelatin (Ejiao 阿胶)

Dragon's blood (Xuejie 血竭)

Dragon's bone (Longgu 龙骨)

Dried ginger (Ganjiang 干姜)

Dried Glauber's salt (Xuanming-fen 玄明粉)

Dried rehmannia (Gandihuang 干地黄)

Earthworm (Dilong 地龙)

Ecklonia (Kunbu 昆布)

Eclipta (Hanliancao 旱莲草)

Elsholtzia (Xiangru 香薷)

Ephedra (Mahuang 麻黄)

Ephedra root (Mahuanggen 麻黄根)

Epimedium (Yinyanghuo 淫羊藿)

Eucommia bark (Duzhong 杜仲)

Eupatorium (Peilan 佩兰)

Euryale seed (Qianshi 芡实)

Evodia fruit (Wuzhuyu 吴茱萸)

Fennel fruit (Xiaohuixiang 小茴香)

Finger citron (Foshou 佛手)

Flattened milkvetch seed (Sha-yuanjili 沙苑蒺藜)

Flavescent sophora root (Kushen 苦参)

Fleece flower root (Heshouwu 何首乌)

Forsythia (Lianqiao 连翘)

Fraxinus (Qinpi 秦皮)

Fresh allium bulb (Shengcongbai 生葱白)

Fresh biota tops (Shengbaiye 生柏叶)

Fresh Chinese angelica root (Shengdangguiwei 生当归尾)

Fresh Chinese mugwort (Sheng-aiye 生艾叶)

Fresh Dolichos flower (Xian Biandouhua 鲜扁豆花)

Fresh ginger (Shengjiang 生姜)

Fresh ginger juice (Shengjiangzhi 生姜汁)

Fresh lotus leaf (Shengheye 生荷叶)

Fresh rehmannia (Shengdihuang

生地黄)

Fringed pink (Qumai 瞿麦)

Fritillary bulb (Beimu 贝母)

Galanga (Gaoliangjiang 高良姜)

Gastrodia tuber (Tianma 天麻)

Genkwa (Yuanhua 芫花)

Germinated barley (Maiya 麦芽)

Ginger juice (Jiangzhi 姜汁)

Ginkgo seed (Baiguo 白果)

Ginseng (Renshen 人参)

Gleditsia spine (Zaojiaoci 皂角刺)

Glehnia (Shashen 沙参)

Green tangerine peel (Qingpi 青皮)

Gypsum (Shigao 石膏)

Hawthorn fruit (Shanzha 山楂)

Hematite (Daizheshi 代赭石)

Honey suckle stem (Rendongteng 忍冬藤)

Honey (Fengmi 蜂蜜)

Houttuynia (Yuxingcao 鱼腥草)

Ignited yellow earth (Zaoxin Huangtu 灶心黄土)

Immature bitter orange (Zhishi 枳实)

Imperata rhizome (Baimaogen 白茅根)

Inula flower (Xuanfuhua 旋复花)

Isatis root (Banlangen 板兰根)

Jujube (Dazao 大枣)

Kansui root (Gansui 甘遂)

Kelp (Haidai 海带)

Large-leaf gentiana (Qinjiao 秦艽)

Ledebouriella root (Fangfeng 防风)

Lepidium seed (Tinglizi 葶苈子)

Licorice (Gancao 甘草)

Light wheat (Fuxiaomai 浮小麦)

Ligusticum (Chuanxiong 川芎)

Ligusticum root (Gaoben 藁本)

Ligustrum fruit (Nüzhenzi 女贞子)

Lindera root (Wuyao 乌药)

Longan aril (Longyanrou 龙眼肉)

Lonicera flower (Jinyinhua 金银花)

Loquat leaf (Pipaye 枇杷叶)

Lotus leaf (Heye 荷叶)

Lotus node (Oujie 藕节)

Lotus seed (Lianzirou 莲子肉)

Lotus stamen (Lianzixu 莲子须)

Lotus stem (Hegeng 荷梗)

Luffa sponge (Sigualuo 丝瓜络)

Lycium fruit (Gouqizi 枸杞子)

Lygodium spores (Haijinsha 海金沙)

Lysimachia (Jinqiancao 金钱草)

Macrostem Onion (Xiebai 薤白)

Madder root (Qiancaogen 茜草根)

Magnetite (Cishi 磁石)

Magnolia bark (Houpo 厚朴)

Magnolia flower (Xinyihua 辛黄花)

Maltose (Yitang 饴糖)

Mastic (Ruxiang 乳香)

Medicated leaven (Shenqu 神曲)

Mentha (Bohe 薄荷)

Mirabilitum (Mangxiao 芒硝)

Morinda root (Bajitian 巴戟天)

Motherwort (Yimucao 益母草)

Moutan bark (Mudanpi 牡丹皮)

Mulberry bark (Sangbaipi 桑白皮)

Mulberry leaf (Sangye 桑叶)

Mulberry mistletoe (Sangjisheng 桑寄生)

Mulberry twig (Sangzhi 桑枝)

Musk (Shexiang 麝香)

Myrrh (Moyao 没药)

Natural indigo (Qingdai 青黛)

Notoginseng powder (Sanqifen 三七粉)

Notopterygium root (Qianghuo 羌活)

Nutmeg (Roudoukou 肉豆蔻)

Ophicalcite (Huaruishi 花蕊石)

Ophiopogon root (Maimendong 麦门冬)

Oriental wormwood (Yinchen 茵陈)

Oryza (Jingmi 粳米)

Oyster shell (Shengmuli 生牡蛎)

Patrinia (Baijiangcao 败酱草)

Peach seed (Taoren 桃仁)

Perilla leaf (Zisuye 紫苏叶)

Perilla seed (Suzi 苏子)

Perilla stem (Sugeng 苏梗)

Peucedanum root (Qianhu 前胡)

Pharbitis seed (Qianniuzi 牵牛子)

Phellodendron (Huangbai 黄柏)

Phragmites stem (Weijing 苇茎)

Picrorrhiza (Huhuanglian 胡黄连)

Pilose asiabell root (Dangshen 党参)

Pinellia tuber (Banxia 半夏)

Plantain seed (Cheqianzi 车前子)

Platycodon (Jiegeng 桔梗)

Polygala root (Yuanzhi 远志)

Polygonatum rhizome (Yuzhu 玉竹)

Polygonatum (Shengweirui 生葳蕤)

Polyporus (Zhuling 猪苓)

Poria (Fuling 茯苓)

Portulaca (Machixian 马齿苋)

Prepared rehmannia (Shudihuang 熟地黄)

Prepared soybean (Dandouchi 淡豆豉)

Prunella spike (Xiakucao 夏枯草)

Psoralea (Buguzhi 补骨脂)

Pubescent angelica root (Duhuo 独活)

Pueraria root (Gegen 葛根)

Puff-ball (Mabo 马勃)

Pulsatilla root (Baitouweng 白头翁)

Pumpkin seed (Nanguazi 南瓜子)

Radish seed (Laifuzi 莱菔子)

Red peony (Chishao 赤芍)

Red poria (Chifuling 赤茯苓)

Red sage root (Danshen 丹参)

Reed root (Lugen 芦根)

Rhinoceros horn (Xijiao 犀角)

Rhubarb (Dahuang 大黄)

Rice soup (Miyin 米饮)

Ricepaper pith (Tongcao 通草)

Round cardamom seed (Baidoukou 白豆蔻)

Rubia root (Qiancao 茜草)

Rush pith (Dengxincao 灯芯草)

Schisandra fruit (Wuweizi 五味子)

Schizonepeta (Jingjie 荆芥)

Schizonepeta spike (Jingjiesui 荆芥穗)

Scorpion (Quanxie 全蝎)

Scrophularia (Xuanshen 玄参)

Scutellaria (Huangqin 黄芩)

Seaweed (Haizao 海藻)

Sea-ear shell (Shijueming 石决明)

Semiaquillegia seed (Zibei Tiankuizi 紫背天葵子)

Sesame seed (Humaren 胡麻仁)

Sichuan chinaberry (Chuanlianzi 川楝子)

Small thistle (Xiaoji 小蓟)

Sophora flower (Huaihua 槐花)

Sophora fruit (Huaijiao 槐角)

Spirodela (Fuping 浮萍)

Stellaria (Yinchaihu 银柴胡)

Stemona root (Baibu 百部)

Swallowwort rhizome (Baiqian 白前)

Swallowwort (Baiwei 白薇)

Sweet wormwood (Qinghao 青蒿)

Talc (Huashi 滑石)

Tangerine seed (Juhe 橘核)

Tea leaf (Chaye 茶叶)

Tendrilled fritillary bulb (Chuanbeimu 川贝母)

Tetrandra root (Fangji 防己)

Thistle (Daji 大蓟)

Tortoise plastron (Guiban 龟板)

Tortoise shell (Biejia 鳖甲)

Tribulus fruit (Baijili 白蒺藜)

Trichosanthes root (Tianhuafen 天花粉)

Trichosanthes (Gualou 瓜蒌)

Trichosanthes skin (Gualoupi 瓜蒌皮)

Tsaoko seed (Caoguoren 草果仁)

Tsaoko (Caoguo 草果)

Turnip seed (Luobozi 萝卜子)

Tussilago flower (Kuandonghua 款冬花)

Typhae pollen (Puhuang 蒲黄)

Uncaria stem (Gouteng 钩藤)

Viola (Zihuadiding 紫花地丁)

Watermelon peel (Xiguapi 西瓜皮)

White atractylodes (Baizhu 白术)

White peony (Baishao 白芍)

White stiff silkworm (Jiangcan 僵蚕)

White wine (Baijiu 白酒)

Wild chrysanthemum (Yejuhua 野菊花)

Wild jujube seed (Suanzaoren 酸枣仁)

Wolfberry bark (Digupi 地骨皮)

Xanthium fruit (Cangerzi 苍耳子)

Yellow rice (Huangmifan 黄米饭)

Zanthoxylum (Shujiao 蜀椒)

Zedoary (Ezhu 莪术)

图书在版编目 (CIP) 数据

实用中医方剂/耿俊英等著
－北京：新世界出版社，1997.6 重印
ISBN 7－80005－118－8

Ⅰ．实… Ⅱ．①耿… Ⅲ．方剂：方书－中国－英文
Ⅳ．R289.2

实 用 中 医 方 剂

耿俊英 等著

＊

新世界出版社出版
（北京百万庄路 24 号）
北京大学印刷厂印刷
中国国际图书贸易总公司发行
（中国北京车公庄西路 35 号）
北京邮政信箱第 399 号　邮政编码 100044
1991 年（英文）第一版　1997 年第三次印刷
ISBN 7－80005－118－8
03200
14－E－2521P